OVERLOOKED: 20/20 IS NOT ENOUGH

ARTHUR S. SEIDERMAN, OD, MA

IN COLLABORATION WITH
BEVERLY BIZUP HAWKINS, RDH, MA

OPTOMETRIC EXTENSION PROGRAM FOUNDATION

Printed in the United States

Published by the Optometric Extension Program Foundation, Inc.

1921 E. Carnegie Ave., 3-L

Santa Ana, CA 92705

Library of Congress Cataloging-in-Publication Data

Seiderman, Arthur.

  Overlooked : 20/20 is not enough / Arthur S. Seiderman ; in collaboration with Beverly Bizup Hawkins. -- 3rd ed.

    p. cm.

  Includes bibliographical references.

  ISBN 978-0-929780-33-7

  1. Visual training. 2. Vision. I. Hawkins, Beverly Bizup. II. Title. III. Title: 20/20 is not enough.

  RE960.S45 2012

  617.7--dc23

                        2012030778

Optometry is the health care profession specifically licensed by state law to prescribe lenses, optical devices and procedures to improve human vision.

Optometry has advanced vision therapy as a unique treatment modality for the development and remediation of the visual process. Effective vision therapy requires extensive understanding of:

- the effects of lenses (including prisms, filters and occluders)
- the variety of responses to the changes produced by lenses
- the various physiological aspects of the visual process
- the pervasive nature of the visual process in human behavior

As a consequence, effective vision therapy requires the supervision, direction and active involvement of the optometrist.

CONTENTS

ACKNOWLEDGEMENTS

My first thanks go to my patients who gave us permission to tell their stories. And, a special thank you to the many professionals who had impact on my professional career: Harold A. Solan, OD, MA, with whom I was associated in practice 1968-71, Jules Abrams, PhD, Stanley Rosner, PhD, Ralph Blanco, PhD, Richard Kavner, OD, Gerry Getman, OD, Robert Kraskin, OD, Robert Wold, OD, Mort Davis, OD, Ralph Schrock, OD, Gerald Senf, PhD, Stanley Kaseno, OD, Richard Apell, OD, John Streff, OD, Lester Glaser, OD, Ann Lucas, PhD, and Phil Schwartz, OD.

For all of the wonderful graphics, we thank Lindsey Sherman.

Friends who supported my efforts always, Ronni and Joel Schrieber, Linda and Leroy M. Kotzen, MD, and Dennis Goodman, MD, who saved my life, I thank you.

Most of all, thanks to my family, Lee, Sonny and Rick Cohen, David and Gretchen Rantanen, Bob Rantanen, Martha and Tay Meister, and Eric and Kristen Rantanen. And, thanks to the prettiest, sweetest, kindest person I have ever known, my wife, Sue.

Arthur S. Seiderman, OD, MA

First I thank Dr. Arthur Seiderman for inviting me to join him in writing this third edition of *20/20 is Not Enough*. It was an honor. I also thank his staff and team of therapists at the Vision Development Center, Rebecca Zimmerman, Kara Garman and Melissa Auker, for inviting me into your workspace to observe and ask questions. All of you were wonderfully supportive and friendly to me.

Second, I thank my mentors. Dr. D. Walter Cohen taught me to value learning, to "give back" and provided the shoulders for me to stand on. Dr. George Claghorn gave the example of writing a book to completion and the knowledge that writing empowers everyone. Dr. Paul Streveler, more than anyone else, gave me scholarly skills, and taught me confidence in writing.

Third, I thank friends and family for putting up with days of absence while my mind was on this book. My husband, Rick, Linds and my dear family, thank you. Thank you Ruth Keller and Nancy Carlson for your unconditional understanding over the years. A special thanks to Sue Seiderman, Dr. Seiderman's lovely wife, who was so kind and warm toward me when I visited their home to work.

Last but not least I wish to thank everyone at OEP, especially Sally Corngold and Bob Williams. You were both wonderful to work with and I could not have completed this project without you.

Beverly Bizup Hawkins, RDH, MA

PREFACE

Two things are necessary to understand this book. First, all people do not perceive the world around them in the same way. Second, as people, we are in large part, products of how we visually perceive and interpret the world around us. 20/20 eyesight is not enough, when vision plays such a large part in who we are and what we become.

What does it mean to have healthy vision? More importantly, what does it mean for vision to foster a healthy mind? There is a difference between having healthy eyes and having healthy vision and this is why *Overlooked: 20/20 is Not Enough* has been written. *Overlooked: 20/20 Is Not Enough* is a book about what goes on in the brain after our eyes deliver light through the retina. It is a book about how the mind makes sense of the world around us, fosters learning, success in our work and good relationships, through the function of vision.

Like the other senses of hearing, taste, smell and touch, vision allows us to experience the world we live in. But eyesight itself is only responsible for a small percent of our experience. Vision, on the other hand, is responsible for the brain's interpretation of light and images the eyes take in. Vision accounts for 80% of our experience with our surroundings and is the primary sense for what makes us human. It is vision, not sight that allows memory, imagination, clairvoyance in thought and perception of the world to take hold.

Vision is more complex than the functioning of each individual eye. Independently, each eye can be healthy and have its health measured, but it is the interaction of both eyes together with the brain, commonly referred to as "binocular vision and perception" that constitutes "vision." When our eyes cannot track or fuse images properly and when each eye is doing its own thing, independent of the other, we end up with some serious problems. These problems confuse the brain and then the brain takes over to problem solve in its own way either by abbreviating the perception or overloading the person.

Ever go into a grocery store and search desperately for something, give up, ask for help, only to find that the item was staring you right in the face. Why didn't your brain register that item? You looked right at it! Well, it is the brain that processes light, images and perceptions so that we can deal with the world around us. When the brain is overloaded, it crops what you take in from the world in ways you never imagine. If our brains do not edit input, we can get overloaded, frustrated and burn out our ability to concentrate. Few people can concentrate bombarded with too much to process.

When the brain is confused or cannot "read" or interpret light waves and images in a meaningful way, the brain problem solves in ways that cause certain symptoms. Some of these symptoms are mild while others are severe and even life threatening. This is the difference between sight and vision and this is why 20/20 is not enough to survive in the high stimulus environment of the 21st century.

Behavioral optometrists are different than general optometrists in that they specialize in brain function as it relates to light that enters the mind through the eyes. Developmental and behavioral optometrists often work closely with occupational therapists, teachers and pediatricians as well as ophthalmologists, psychologists, reading specialists and optometrists. Earlier books, such as Dr. Richard Kavner's, *Total Vision* and *Your Child's Vision*, have wonderful descriptions of the aforementioned.

As already mentioned, vision, unlike sight, is the foundation of memory, imagination, perception and most of all learning. To read and comprehend written material as well as "to read faces and body language" we need a strong visual system that delivers images through the retina to the brain with the right shape and focus, so the brain can engage us with accurate interpretations.

What are we looking at? If we see partial shapes, words that swim, distorted depth or double images, the brain develops thoughts and feelings that are just as garbled. Many can relate to dyslexic type symptoms, reversed letters, reversed words and numbers. What if someone's smile is reversed in someone's eyes? We all assume that we see what others see and that others see what we see. But this is simply not true! Very few people see the world as identical to another human being, metaphorically and physiologically. *Overlooked: 20/20 is Not Enough* is written to clarify these statements and to logically explain how these slips in understanding can happen.

As you can imagine by now, without healthy vision, perception of reality can be quite altered. Since the first publishing of *20/20 is Not Enough* in 1990, the academic community has discovered many more connections between vision and personality, vision and cognitive differences as well as the connection between vision and ADD/ADHD, autism and addictive behavior. For these reasons, this updated version of this all time classic book on vision therapy includes three new very important chapters. One chapter is dedicated to attention deficit spectrum disorders. A second new chapter is on autism spectrum disorders while the final new chapter is on drug addiction patterns.

This is an exciting time for vision therapy, a specialized field of eye care, historically rich in problem solving the multifunctional nature of vision as the window to the brain. When the first edition of *20/20 is Not Enough* was published, it was authored by Arthur Seiderman, OD, Steven Marcus, OD, and David Hapgood. Groundwork was caringly laid for parents, teachers, athletes and health care professionals as well as for youngsters with poor reading and learning ability. The book was written to enable the general public to grasp an understanding of the powerful relation between the organs of sight and the functioning of the mind. As with any seminal work, its contents were heavily challenged and over the decades that followed, Dr. Seiderman's work repeatedly proves to have opened doors for those who needed to improve accuracy in diagnosis and treatment of various types of problems that relate to vision and behavior.

The first edition of *20/20 is Not Enough* encouraged awareness of the synergistic aspects of eye and brain function and introduced the notion that vision therapy can be a valuable tool in treating visual and behavioral problems, thus improving overall human functioning, particularly at school and at work.

Since the first edition, thousands of people have been helped, so much so that there are numerous books on the subject of vision therapy, many of which were inspired by those who were helped. There are websites, self help software, gadgets and games designed to stimulate brain function as it relates to vision. Organizations and professional associations dealing with vision therapy have flourished and more recently, companies that manufacture anti-aging and brain development software for old and young alike, have adopted the basic tenets that emerged from the early work of the pioneers in vision therapy. The *Los Angeles Times* published an article on June 22, 2009, titled "The Key to 3-D Vision." (http://articles.latimes.com/2009/ jun/22/opinion/oe-barry22. Last accessed: July 10, 2012)

In this article, Dr. Susan Barry, professor of neurobiology at Mt. Holyoke College, and author of the book, *Fixing My Gaze,* relays to readers her personal experience with crossed eyes as a baby. Three surgeries appeared to have corrected her problem, but only served to further mask her vision impairment. After the surgeries, her eyes may have looked like they were straight, but she was still stereoblind. The straightness only served to further mask a serious underlying visual impairment. According to Dr. Barry, this type of overlooked visual impairment condemns children to see in only two dimensions and can go unrecognized for years. Worse yet, it often is mistaken for other stigmatizing disorders. She spent a childhood, nervous and confused in cluttered environments because she could not see space between objects and could not have fun when other kids her age were being entertained.

The benefits of vision therapy are no longer a mystery and have become quite a hub of help for learning disabilities of all kinds and for those with compromised lifestyles due to partial vision. Problems that include poor reading, poor comprehension, attention span, concentration deficits and pain from headaches generally lead to feelings of failure, anger, boredom and even delinquency. Deeply rooted in the brain, our eyes have the ability to teach us to develop confidence, pay attention, work smarter and interact well with others.

In 2009, the NAACP made a ruling that vision therapy helped reduce delinquency, curb the crime rate and improve rehabilitation. (http://www.prnewswire.com/ news-releases/naacp-passes-resolution-on-optometric-vision-therapy-62608562. html. Last accessed: July 10, 2012) The ruling calls attention to the role that vision therapy can play in reducing the high rate of recidivism among our youth. The ruling also aggressively asserts " action must be taken to include Vision Therapy in all re-entry programs for formerly incarcerated persons."

At the 100th Anniversary Convention of the NAACP held in New York City, optometric vision therapy was endorsed as a potential way to help prisoners become productive members of society. Vision therapy was also recognized as having a positive impact on academic performance, preventing high school dropout as well as juvenile delinquency.

Overlooked and untreated vision problems in the United States are a serious public health issue. Undetected and undertreated vision problems are an issue of access to preventive information and an issue of access to care. In some cases the lack of access to care also reflects a lack of professional integrity. These untreated problems affect all of us, even those who already have good vision. Study after study has proven that without help, youths with vision problems have poor work performance, poor school performance, difficulty concentrating and lower paying jobs. Access to vision therapy is a class issue, is both an inner city as well as a rural issue. Vision therapy is an educational issue, an economic issue and a safety issue.

This updated and newly named edition of *Overlooked: 20/20 is Not Enough* builds upon the foundation established in the first edition; accurate information on vision therapy in a self-help style format written for adults and parents of children struggling to make sense of the world that requires accurate vision and the ability to comfortably sustain concentration.

Beverly Bizup Hawkins, RDH, MA

CHAPTER 1
VISION IS LEARNED

"It is a terrible thing to see and have no vision." Helen Keller

Optometrists, as the primary health care professionals for vision, have a long history of caring about how well people can see to read, and how that may affect learning. (Flax 1968, Flax 1972, Morrison, Giordano, Nagy 1977, Solan 1989, Solan, Ciner 1989, Solan 1990) Whenever people have trouble concentrating to read, it is critical to check for visual insufficiency before labeling the difficulty as a "learning disability" or "attention deficit disorder." This is especially true for children and it is usually the teachers who are the first to pick up that there is a problem. In fact, the classic sign of a binocular vision problem is a short attention span and inability to concentrate.

Being a productive individual in society is increasingly dependent upon good reading skills. (National Institutes of Health, 1985) Populations with undetected vision-related reading problems are an increasing public health concern, too. (McAlister et al. 1996 Smith et al. 2000) *Overlooked: 20/20 is Not Enough* is written for parents, kids, clinicians, teachers and public health policy makers. It is a book about what it means to have a comprehensive visual exam that goes well beyond the brief 20/20 Snellen Test. *Overlooked* is a book about how vision relates to learning ability, cognitive function and brain chemistry.

Imagine seeing double but thinking everyone sees the same. Imagine words that jump or disappear. Imagine letters in mirror or word reversed images such as d/b, p/q, 9/6 or order reversals making you see "was" instead of "saw" and "dog" instead of "god." Sounds confusing, doesn't it? Well, it is.

In order to have success at reading you need good recognition between letters. You need to be able to picture in your mind what is happening when you read a story. You also need to be able to retain and recall details of what you read. These latter two concepts are referred to as reading comprehension and retention.

People can have perfect 20/20 eyesight and still have serious visual problems like those just described because each eye is working independently and not working together as a team. Working together as a team is often referred to as "binocular vision." Lack of teamwork of each individual eye can cause serious distortion in thinking and learning along with the inability to sustain visual concentration. Consequences of poor eye coordination seriously affect a person's perception and interpretation of the world around them. When vision is distorted, thinking is distorted. Visual perception relates to how an individual processes information received through the visual system. When visual perception is distorted, thinking is distorted.

Such problems can hamper learning, hinder productivity, and even cause accidents. Socially, vision problems can be the root of discord within a family, causing a great deal of anguish, frustration and anger. Such problems exist more often than you might think. They often run in families, and insidiously go undetected and untreated because an eye exam might have only checked for a 20/20 criteria.

Correcting visual "processing" abnormalities requires the expert help of a doctor who specializes in vision. Eye doctors who are educated to diagnose and treat visual insufficiencies are usually optometrists with special certification in optometric vision therapy. This type of special eye doctor is also called a behavioral or developmental optometrist due to their highly specialized training in how the brain organizes and understands the input of light from each eye to the brain. Their expertise further incorporates how visual processing by the brain, relates to cognition, brain function and human behavior.

In order to understand why main stream clinicians miss many visual problems, it may be helpful to think of behavioral optometrists as vision psychologists. Unlike traditional eye doctors who deal with diseases of the eye and eye surgery, behavioral optometrists are also trained to help the mind's processing of information and improve awareness of the world that the eyes take in through rays of light. Simply put, in the world of the optometrist who is trained in vision therapy; *20/20 is not enough.*

If you sense that something in you or your child's life is just not right; that there is something wrong and you can't put your finger on it, chances are you may be dealing with vision problems. And, it may be time to seek a complete visual exam by a qualified optometrist certified in vision therapy. Professional organizations that provide a clinician locator service along with information, research findings and patient handouts are the Optometric Extension Program Foundation, www.oepf. org, the College of Optometrists in Vision Development, www.covd.org, and the Neuro-Optometric Rehabilitation Association, www.nora.cc.

Just as you may have two healthy hands, few people are able to sit down and play the piano without lessons and practice. Learning to play piano involves coordinating both hands to perform together while simultaneously doing something else, such as concentrating on the music. Well, eyes are no different. Both eyes need the same coordination training in order to perform well enough to enable the mind to focus, function and concentrate. Some people are better equipped at having everyday activities foster the coordination needed to thrive visually. Others however are not as lucky and need professional help. Often genetic factors play a role in total visual functioning and problems that children have in school start to become familiar to parents as they reflect on their childhood struggles. Poor vision can run in families.

One of the main tools for efficient reading comprehension and test taking is binocular and perceptual function. When visual concentration cannot be sustained reading comprehension becomes limited, and the lack of sustainability is often due to binocular disparity.

Binocular vision impairments are more common than you may think. Research findings published by Hokada (1985) found that 21% of a normal population demonstrated both symptoms and clinical findings of binocular vision impairments. This means that about one in every five people have problems with vision that could be helped with vision therapy. In a reading disabled population 73% exhibit binocular and/ or perceptual dysfunction. (Seiderman 1980)

Since both eyes sit separately, they do not look at objects from the same angle and depth. Each eye sees its own image of the same object, and is dependent upon the other eye and the brain to bring the object into focus as one. When the eyes and brain have not learned how to do this, the result can be double vision and differences in depth perception. Without synchronized binocular vision, just 20 minutes of close work (within 14 to 20 inches for an adult) is enough time to create a level of eyestrain that affects concentration, frustration, loss of patience and even anger.

With children, 5-10 minutes of trying to read at a distance of 6-12 inches, with double vision is enough to cause the level of eyestrain that affects concentration. For such a child, the common consequence, whether subconscious or as a defense mechanism, is to avoid reading. In other words they just can't do it, so they avoid it.

Vision therapy helps people develop quality vision and improve concentration. It is an extension of brain function. There is extensive knowledge gained every year on the relation between vision and cognitive performance, particularly learning. The chapters ahead explain how to reduce eyestrain as well as headaches and other symptoms of eyestrain. Vision therapy helps to improve concentration, enhance peripheral vision and depth perception as well as improve visual reaction time.

Visual disorders are integrally related to learning disabilities including visual perception problems in children with attention deficit disorder (ADD) and attention deficit hyperactivity disorder (ADHD), as well as autism and problems with certain types of addictive behavioral patterns.

By now you should be gaining an understanding that training the visual system for maximum function is important. The world of technology asks our eyes to perform at levels never before expected of human vision. The need for glasses was never so great before the 20th century when more and more of our daily living demanded close small work and visual focus that was previously unnatural. We have made an adaptation here due to increased need for academic performance and computer usage, which has, in turn, increased the incidence of nearsightedness. This is the result of an accommodative convergence system, meaning that the eyes must turn inward to work at close range.

Of course not all problems in the world are vision related, but with nearly 80% of human functioning relying on good vision (Farrald 1973) and with visual memory existing as a critical aspect of learning, a comprehensive visual exam starts to take precedence in overall health and potential for thriving. Vision therapy helps people in a variety of ways, with research solidifying the facts. Vision therapy takes time and patience, and success rates are well documented when delivered by qualified optometrists working together with reading and learning specialists or occupational therapists and psychologists. It is not, however, a panacea. Vision therapy is a carefully studied application of a holistic approach to the marriage of both eyes with the functioning of the brain and the mind's eye. For this reason it is also referred to as "neurovisual therapy."

Vision therapy aims at correcting binocular vision, oculomotor visual processing, and perceptual disorders. Vision therapy is especially helpful to those who suffer from double vision, visually-related headaches as well as eyestrain. Others find sports vision enhancement therapy to be invaluable in maximizing athletic performance with improved visual reaction time, eye-hand coordination and visual tracking skills.

Again, because the emphasis on 20/20 eyesight tests, many treatable vision problems go untreated. Functional visual problems may be missed during a routine eye exam. Anger and hostility are often consequences of untreated visual problems because the visual cortex of the brain simply gets overloaded. The result is often manifested in frustration and emotional problems.

Patterns of visually-related anger and frustration, attention deficit (ADD) and attention deficit hyperactivity (ADHD) disorders, have been linked to binocular and visual perceptual problems. For all of these reasons it is important for parents, teachers and health care professionals to be able to screen and identify children who may need referrals for appropriate help for functional and perceptual visual problems.

There are three types of eyecare professionals. *Ophthalmologists* are eye doctors who attend medical school first and later choose a two-year residency in ophthalmology. Ophthalmologists are best known as surgeons and doctors who treat diseases of the eye.

In contrast, the optometric physician is an eye doctor commonly known as an *optometrist*. Optometrists are eye care professionals with the broadest educational background in total vision as it relates to human behavior. Optometrists earn a four-year undergraduate degree followed by another four years of graduate study at a school of optometry. Many further their study beyond the doctorate by choosing a postgraduate residency specialty.

One such specialty where a physician of optometry may acquire expert knowledge is oculomotor control as it relates to cognitive perceptual skills, spatial perception, visual memory and learning. This type of optometrist will often work closely with occupational therapists, psychologists, pediatricians, teachers, reading specialists, speech and language pathologists and children diagnosed with developmental or behavioral learning problems. This type of optometrist is called an *optometric vision therapy physician*. For an optometric vision therapist, it is no coincidence that the phrase "I see" means "I understand" or that "20/20 is not enough."

The third type of eye care specialist is the *optician*. Opticians are health care professionals who design, fit and dispense lenses for the correction of a person's eyesight.

Again, seeking a complete vision evaluation from a credentialed optometrist (certified fellow in vision therapy) is important particularly since vision therapy specialists are often not found in the neighborhood directory. It is important to contact a *certified fellow* and drive the distance it takes to be fruitful in your endeavors to solve visual problems. In order to find a credentialed vision therapy optometrist, contact the Optometric Extension Program (www.oepf.org.) , College of Optometrists in Vision Development (www.covd.org) or and the Neuro-Optometric Rehabilitation Association (www.nora.cc).

THE SNELLEN TEST

The standard eye test is familiar to most everyone. You sit in a chair and look across the room at a chart on the wall with letters and numbers in decreasing size, starting with the big E. The eye doctor asks you to read as many lines as you can from the top down. If your performance is below normal, the eye doctor asks you to look through lenses until you can see normally in each individual eye. In fact, the prescription for correction is written in two parts, one for the left and one for the right eye. Your eyes are further examined for diseases of the eye such as glaucoma or macular degeneration and then you leave with your prescription for a pair of glasses. Sometimes the diagnosis may reveal need for further medical treatment or surgery

What did that examination reveal? The chart on the wall, known as the Snellen chart (for its inventor, the Dutch ophthalmologist Herman Snellen), has remained essentially unchanged since the time of our Civil War. It was designed to find out if a child can see what a teacher is writing on the blackboard. It doesn't do much more than that. Discerning letters on a wall 20 feet away is not how most of us use our eyes.

The Snellen test does not answer the most important questions. It does not show if a child having trouble in grade school is visually equipped to read. Reading is a continuing process of seeking information at close range that is far different from making out the letters on the chart. It tells us still less about whether an older student can handle the much greater reading demands of high school or college. The test does not tell us if the vision of an accountant, dentist or data entry specialist is suited to doing visually intensive close work all day long.

It does not tell us if a driver has the visual reaction time to see a car approaching from the side so he can hit the brakes in order to avoid an accident or the depth perception to tell how far away it is. It does not tell us if a young athlete's visual reaction time is good enough to save him from serious injury. This applies to all activities that hold safety risks.

The traditional Snellen Test treats each eye as if it were an independent entity, and corrective lenses are prescribed for each eye independently. Nothing in that prescription necessarily fosters dual, simultaneous use of the eyes together as the whole organ of vision. People are binocular beings. Binocular vision, the product of the two eyes working together, is what enables us to see in three dimensions, and is essential to everything we do all day long.

As the traditional doctor sees it, there is nothing he or she can do for the patient beyond prescribing glasses and treating disease. The traditional eye exam using the Snellen Test does not answer the question: "Can this person be helped to use vision more effectively?" This is one of the reasons that many visual disorders go undiagnosed rather than be easily treated.

Much is now known about how people can care for their eyes in order to minimize the effects of intensive close work, and much also is known about the beneficial effects of good nutrition. Traditional eye doctors often do not supply patients with any of that information; it's not part of the generic eye exam.

Practitioners who restrict the eye exam to eyeball function are only examining sight and are not including an evaluation of total vision. The difference is crucial. Sight occurs in the eyes alone. Vision is the interplay between the eyes and the brain. Humans are born with sight, but vision is learned. In our first days of life we can "see," but we cannot see in any meaningful sense because our brain has not learned how to see. We do not yet have vision.

By now you may be coming to the correct conclusion that the Snellen Chart is just the beginning. Both eyes must be examined working together not treated as independent entities. The two lenses prescribed for the glasses are just that, two separate, nonintegrated prescriptions.

People are binocular beings. Binocular vision, the product of the eyes working together, is what enables us to see in 3-D and is essential to almost everything we do all day long. As an ophthalmologist may understand it, there is nothing more that can be done for the patient beyond the prescription for the glasses or treating disease if it is found.

Vision as an integrated whole with the mind is not a new idea. Plato's ideal of vision was that it was a ray of light that we beam out from our minds to collect the images we see. As a metaphor, that is a pretty good description of what happens. Plato further emphasized how the mind interprets incorrectly when vision is flawed. There is no better illustration of Plato's deep concern for education as it relates to

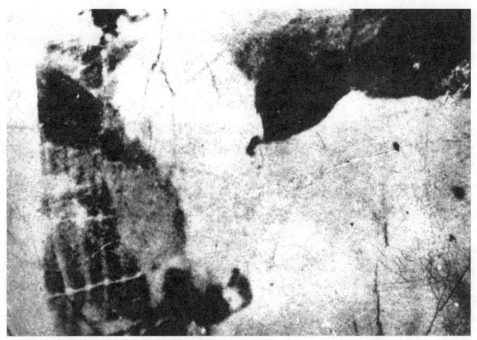

SIGHT AND VISION

What do you see? At first glance this photo seems to show only meaningless shapes. Vision is the process by which the brain organizes the information it receives from the eyes to give it meaning. Once that occurs, this picture will never again look to you as it did at first. The photo shows a cow and is known as the "Renshaw Cow." (Photo courtesy of the Optometric Extension Program Foundation)

vision than that of the "Allegory of the Cave" from *The Republic*. In the parable, Plato asks us to imagine trying to interpret images cast on the wall of a cave without being able to see the actual objects, only their shadows. You only see the shadows in front of you and not the objects behind you brought to life by a small fire, which causes them to dance about.

The prisoners, as they are called, can talk between themselves but are dependent upon what they see on the wall to assume what is real. Shadows seen on the wall are the only reality they experience and understanding of the world is open to individual interpretation and assumption. Reality is altered as you can well imagine. Plato's "Allegory of the Cave" is a metaphor for sight, perception and knowledge acquired without full vision.

What is important to remember is that not all eye care professionals do a thorough visual examination including binocular vision and perception testing. Many just measure whether or not you can see the dancing shadows clearly. For this reason it is important for you to ask questions, be open-minded and trust the optometrist knowledgeable in all aspects of vision development. A good place to start is by referring to the following website: www.helpaddvisiontherapy.com

The picture we see as we look out at the world is not in our eyes but only in our brain. That is where we give meaning to the eyes' messages. To take just one example, the eyes cannot interpret size, and so a fist held at arm's length appears bigger on the retina than a building half a mile away. It is the brain that, on the basis of what it has learned in the past, makes order of that jumble. The brain decides that the building is, in fact, larger than the fist. By directing the eyes' attention, the brain decides what information it will have them collect, then decides what small part of that information it will notice and what meaning it will give to the information. That is why two people whose eyes have registered exactly the same messages may, and usually will, perceive what is out there quite differently.

Plato was essentially right: the brain reaches out and imposes its individual meaning on the collection of messages it receives from the eyes. Each of us creates our own visual world and each is unique. This is vision, and without sight the image in the eye has no useful purpose.

When we say, "I see a cow," we refer to our vision, not our sight, because our eyes don't know what a cow is. The brain scans the messages sent by the eyes to estimate size and shape, compares the result with images stored in visual memory, and concludes that what is out there is what it knows to be a cow. At the same time the brain matches those pictures to its memory of language to summon the spoken and perhaps written word that means, "cow."

Vision is the window of the mind, the primary way we perceive the world around us. We are visual beings; sight has become overwhelmingly the most important of our senses. About 80% of the information that reaches us comes through our eyes. The volume of information collected by our eyes is astonishing. Each eye sends the brain a billion messages during every waking second. Together the eyes send twice as many messages as the entire rest of the body, including all the other senses. It was not always so. As our species has evolved, we have used our vision to extend our perception of the world past the reach of more limited senses. Our ancestors had more need than we of the sense of smell, and species farther back on the evolutionary path depended primarily on other senses.

Today, vision is more dominant than it was in the past, so much so that visual messages often overload the other senses. Our eyes send 430 times as many messages to the brain as do our ears. That is why we close our eyes when we listen to music. The sound is no different, yet we hear the music as fuller and richer when we shut out the overpowering messages of sight. Similarly, we often close our eyes to appreciate taste or smell. Our very language reveals the dominance of sight in such metaphors as "look into" and "foresight" and "vision" itself. We say, "I see" to mean, "I understand," while, if they could speak, a bloodhound would no doubt say "I smell" and a bat would surely say, "I hear."

Our dominant sense so shapes our perception of the world around us, and therefore our behavior in that world, that in a large measure we are what we see, not what we touch or hear or smell. Our personalities are influenced by our visual perceptions: differing kinds of vision make for different kinds of people. Nearsighted people tend more than others to be loners, meticulous, shy, introverted. The outgoing personality is more likely to be farsighted. Because we learn vision in childhood, varying circumstances in the earliest years may make for different ways of seeing and so produce somewhat different personalities

Today, the nature of modern life has placed an unprecedented stress on the dominant sense of vision by asking our eyes to do work for which they were not designed. Most people find that their eyes, when relaxed and free of any immediate task, tend to be more comfortable gazing off into the far distance than looking at something close at hand. There is good evolutionary reason for this. Distant vision was what mattered most to our remote ancestors. The necessities of life for which they searched, game and fruit and nuts, had to be discerned when they were far away. So did the enemies they had to avoid. Those among our ancestors who saw best at a distance were the likeliest to survive; they were the fittest. When, much later, our ancestors took up farming, they still depended mainly on distant vision. True, they did some close-up work—making tools, for example—but they did not need to see in fine detail, nor did they spend most of their waking day at it. And nobody read anything at all.

These realities remained essentially unchanged until recently. We invented writing, but only a minority acquired this new skill, and even of those only a very few spent their working days reading and writing. That was true of most societies (and is still true of some) until well into the 20th century, which, on the scale of human evolution, was not even yesterday but more like an hour ago.

Now, in modern society, and for the first time ever, the majority of people earn their living at tasks they perform less than an arm's length from their eyes. We spend our working days with our eyes focused at that short distance. For most people, their work involves reading—that is, interpreting small symbols on a printed page or more likely, on a computer screen. Schooling, the gateway to success in modern life, which occupies us from age five usually into our 20s, is virtually synonymous with reading. What's asked of us, moreover, is not just knowing how to read, but how to read rapidly and accurately and for hours on end. If we can't do that, we'll fall behind the pack.

Spending our days working intensively at close range puts a heavy strain on eyes designed to search for distant game. Eyes adapt by becoming myopic (nearsighted). Indeed, the prevalence of myopia is one of the surest signs of modernity. If half the people you see on the street are wearing corrective lenses, you can be sure you are walking around in an advanced society. For the evidence is by now overwhelming that, contrary to what is still widely believed, myopia is in most cases developed rather than inherited. Among the many studies that make this point, two are particularly dramatic. In a survey of Eskimo families, among 130 children who were illiterate, only two were nearsighted, while of their peers who attended school, 65%

were myopic. The difference was not inherited, for the parents and grandparents of both groups were equally farsighted. In Japan before the Second World War, the rate of myopia approximated that in the United States. During the war years education was neglected, and at war's end it was discovered that myopia among school age children had dropped to half its prewar rate. After the war Japan recovered, education resumed and so did the incidence of myopia. Overall, epidemiological studies show that a family history of myopia and close-up work are the two strongest risk factors.(Saw et al. 1996)

Nearsightedness is only one of the effects of modern life on our visual system. Given the strains of functioning in contemporary society, it should come as no surprise that a great many of us have problems with our vision. The standard estimate is that 70% of Americans have less than adequate vision. This means that a majority of us get less than full use from our vital, dominant sense, the sense through which we primarily interpret what is around us. We are missing anywhere from a little to a great deal of what is going on, and we are responding accordingly.

Vision problems show themselves in many ways. For some, the effects may be mainly physical: the eyestrain, headache, and exhaustion experienced by people who do close work all day. For others, faulty vision manifests itself in missed opportunities, in a life that could be better. They could feel healthier than they do. They could do better in their work, be more successful in their careers, if their visual system functioned better than it does.

At first glance, visual problems may seem entirely personal, but in fact an individual's faulty vision can affect the lives of others in several ways. We all know about the huge numbers killed or maimed each year on our highways. All states require an eye examination in order to obtain a license, but in almost all cases it consists of nothing more than a test of distant vision on the familiar Snellen chart. Other visual skills essential to safe driving, such as depth perception, peripheral vision, and visual reaction time, are rarely tested in the United States (though some are tested in Europe). Surely many lives would be saved if all of us could see as well to drive as we can to read the letters on a motionless wall chart. Some children who fail in school because of visual problems will in time drop out and may even become delinquent.

Brian Mohney, MD, of the Mayo Clinic published results of a study (Mohney 2008) in the journal, *Pediatrics*. The results showed that children with divergent strabismus were three times more likely to develop a psychiatric disorder than children with normal eye alignment. Also proven was that patients with intermittent divergent strabismus were more likely to have mental health disorders and thoughts of suicide or homicide.

Athletes and sports fans are of course vigorous critics of the visual skills of officials. A Peter Arno cartoon of many years ago shows a minister rising in the stands to bellow in righteous anger: "Thou hast eyes but thou seest not!" That minister would no doubt feel vindicated by a study made of 40 umpires and referees by Dr. Seiderman. In the study, (Seiderman 1980) Dr. Seiderman found that a surprisingly large proportion of referees and umpires studied, lacked normal vision. One quarter of them failed to score 20/20 on the eye chart. Interestingly enough, a larger number had inadequate depth perception, a skill that is seldom tested, yet is essential to such work. Some officials had glasses but did not wear them at work for fear the fans would laugh at them. Visual problems can have far more serious consequences for the athletes themselves. Boxers and football players have died from injuries they could have avoided had they worked to speed up their visual reaction time.

In later chapters we will meet a variety of people who found another way to improve their vision. A few examples will illustrate the range of possibilities among those who have less than perfect vision. At one extreme is Peter B, an amateur race car driver. He had no problem with his eyes. His vision was already excellent, better than that of most people, and he did not need to wear glasses. "But I wanted that last one percent, because of the difference it could make on the racetrack," he said.

Brendan M and Shari M were at the other extreme. Brendan's visual disabilities prevented him from learning to read, and Shari's kept her from reading at the high school level. They were among the great number of American schoolchildren who suffer from a learning disability, or perform far below their potential, partly or wholly because of an untreated visual disorder. For both Brendan and Shari the problem was that their eyes did not work properly together as a team, so they found it painful to read for any length of time. But since they had passed the eye-chart test, their visual needs went unnoticed for too long. Both Brendan and Shari were headed toward failure in school and, almost certainly, in adult life.

Gretchen S's life was changed drastically for the worse in her 40s when the onset of double vision not only forced her to give up her work but also made such routine activities as reading and driving suddenly difficult. Two eye operations left her no better off than before.

Two other examples fall between these extremes. David H, an editor, was one of many people who are successful at doing intensive close work despite a moderate visual handicap. His disorder manifested itself in fidgetiness and lack of concentration at his desk, and eyes that felt tired by mid afternoon. He did his work, and did it well, but not as well or as quickly as he could have: he scored perhaps a B- rather than his potential B+. Libby K's visual disorder was fairly severe, but in compensation her life as an adult made relatively mild demands on her vision. Her trouble manifested itself in mishaps during routine tasks. She bumped into kitchen cabinets and she drove her car up on the curb too often for these things to be merely accidental, and she didn't read even the newspaper because it was too much work.

These six stories all have happy endings, as we will see in greater detail in later chapters. Peter is doing better on the racetrack. "Now time moves more slowly in a race," he says. "My car and the other cars the whole track seems to be moving in slow motion." Brendan, who could not learn to read in second grade, won a reading prize the next year and eventually went on to graduate from an Ivy League college. Shari who did poorly in her freshman year, got A's and B's as a sophomore. "I love school now," she said that second year. "My friends think I'm smart."

Gretchen's vision is getting steadily better, despite the effects of two needless operations. David, the editor, gets more and better work done each day with less discomfort; even his tennis has improved within the limits of the possible. Libby finds she gets through her days far more comfortably. "I'm not so nervous now," she says. "I don't bump into things."

What made the difference is the process known as vision therapy.

EVALUATING YOUR VISION

What follows are two sets of questions designed to help the reader judge the state of his or her own vision. The first set of 12 questions describes major signs of a problem in one's vision. If you answer "yes" to any of these first 10 questions, you would be wise to get a full examination by an eye doctor who tests the skills of vision as well as sight.

- Do your eyes hurt?
- Do you see double?
- Does your vision blur when you look to the distance, or when you are doing close work?
- Do your eyes water a lot?
- Do your eyes get very bloodshot?
- Do you see more clearly with one eye than the other?
- Do you get headaches after intense visual activities such as reading or driving?
- Do you ever see flashes of light?
- Is part of your field of vision missing in one or both eyes?
- Do you feel dizzy or sick to your stomach after intensive close work or activity?
- Do you have difficulty concentrating?
- Does your mind tend to wander?

The following, much longer list, is of less severe signs of possible visual problems. We believe you should consider a full visual examination if you answer "yes" to between five and 10 of these questions. If you answer "yes" to more than ten questions, then we suggest you promptly seek such an examination.

- Do your eyes tire quickly when you are reading or working at a video display terminal?
- Does your comprehension tend to decrease the longer you read?

- Do you confuse similar words or letters while reading?
- Do you skip words while reading?
- Do you lose your place while reading?
- Do you read slowly?
- Do you read word by word?
- Do you often have to reread a line you've just read?
- Do you sound words aloud or move your lips silently when reading, ?
- Do you use your finger or a marker to keep your place while reading or writing?
- Do you have difficulty remembering what you've read?
- Does your mind wander when you're reading?
- Do you avoid reading?
- Do you hold your head close to what you're reading or writing?
- Do you turn your head so you are using only one eye?
- Do you turn your head a great deal while reading or working at a computer?
- Do you rub your eyes frequently during or after reading or working at a computer?
- Do you tilt your head to the side to read?
- Do you close or cover one eye?
- Do you write neatly but very slowly?
- Do you have trouble with spelling?
- Do you often reverse letters, words, or numbers?
- Are you restless when working at your desk?
- Does your distance vision blur when you look up from close work?
- Do you lose visual clarity when you concentrate?
- Do you do poorly on standardized tests?
- Do you have difficulty with written directions or instructions?
- Do you dislike tasks requiring sustained visual attention?
- Do lights bother your eyes?
- Do you avoid close work?
- Do you feel unusually tired after you complete a visual task?
- Do you feel nervous, irritable, restless, or frustrated after sustained visual concentration?
- Do you learn better from listening than from seeing?
- When concentrating do you tend to lose awareness of your surroundings?

- Do you daydream a lot?
- Do you frequently trip or stumble?
- Do you have trouble threading a needle?
- Do you find it difficult to see another person's point of view?
- Do you find it difficult to visualize an action and its consequences before you take it?
- Do you blink a lot?
- Do you have frequent sties?
- Do you avoid eye contact when talking to people?
- Do you find it hard to remember people's faces?
- Do you find it difficult to use binoculars?
- Do you feel uncomfortable in a crowded area with a lot of movement such as a shopping mall, terminal, or department store?
- Do you have trouble reading a map?
- Do you tailgate when driving?
- Do you have trouble judging distance while parking?
- Do you find night driving difficult?
- Do you get carsick?
- Are eye-hand-coordination sports such as tennis, racquetball or baseball difficult for you?
- Are eye-body-coordination activities such as dancing difficult for you?

REFERENCES

Farrald RR, Shamber RG 1973. A diagnostic and prescriptive technique: a mainstream approach to identification, assessment and amelioration of learning disabilities. Sioux Falls, S.D:Adapt Press.

Flax N 1972. The eye and learning disabilities. J Am Optom Assoc 43:612.

Flax N 1972. The eye and learning disabilities. J School Health 44: 83–85.

Flax N 1968. Visual function in dyslexia. Am J Optom Arch Am Acad Optom 45:574-87.

Hokoda SC 1985. General binocular dysfunctions in an urban optometry clinic. J Am Optom Assoc 56:560-3.

Mayo Clinic 2008. Eye Divergence in Children Triples Risk of Mental Illness. November 26, 2008. http://www.mayoclinic.org/news2008-rst/5103.html.

McAlister WH, Garzia RP, Nicholson SB 1996. Public health issues and reading disability. In: Garzia RP, ed. Vision and Reading. St. Louis, MO: Mosby-Year Book.

Mohney BG, McKenzie JA, Capo JA, Nusz KJ, Mrazek D, Diehl NN, 2008. Mental illness in young adults who had strabismus as children. Pediatrics 122:1033–8.

Morrison FJ, Giordano B, Nagy J 1977. Reading disability: An informational processing analysis. Science 196:77-9.

National Institutes of Health. Becoming a Nation of Readers: The report of the Commission on Reading 1985. Washington, DC: National Institute of Health.

Saw SM, Katz J, Schein OD, Chew SJ, Chan TK 1996. *Epidemiology of Myopia. Epidemiologic Reviews. Johns Hopkins University School of Hygiene and Public Health:18.*

Seiderman AS 1980. *Optometric vision therapy: Results of a demonstration project with a learning disabled population. J Am Optom Assoc 51:489-93.*

Smith M, Mikulecky L, Kibby MW, Dreher MJ, Dole JA 2000. *What will be the demands of literacy in the workplace in the next millennium? Reading Res Qtly 35:378–83.*

Solan HA, Ciner EB 1989. *Visual perception and learning: issues and answers. J Am Optom Assoc 60:457-60.*

Solan HA 1979. *Learning disabilities: The role of the developmental optometrist. J Am Optom Assoc 50:1259-65.*

Solan HA 1990. *Learning disabilities. In: Rosenbloom AA, Morgan MM, eds. Principles and Practice of Pediatric Optometry. Philadelphia: J.B. Lippincott.*

CHAPTER 2
VISION THERAPY:
FINDING HELP

It is not surprising that many people are unfamiliar with vision therapy. Not all optometrists are trained in behavioral optometry, or become certified fellows in vision therapy. Ophthalmologists, as experts at surgery and diseases of the eye, have less training in brain plasticity as it relates to total functional vision. Perhaps, a neurologist, psychologist or occupational therapist would recognize the need for vision therapy faster than other specialists since visual perceptual deficiencies relate to brain function and behavioral outcomes.

Teachers, health care professionals and parents are encouraged to take the information in this book seriously, and assertively engage in dialogues with students and parents whom they feel may have poor vision. Increasing education and awareness of ignored health problems are ethical responsibilities. To do otherwise is a form of neglect.

Once again, the categories of eye practitioners can be confusing. Optometrists, who are graduates of a four year post college professional school of optometry, are primary health care providers who prescribe glasses and examine the eyes for disease. In some states, optometrists are also licensed to treat certain types of disease, and perform some surgery. Ophthalmologists, who belong to a medical specialty, are trained to treat disease and perform surgery; they may or may not prescribe glasses. Opticians make the glasses prescribed by others. The term "oculist," once applied to both optometrists and ophthalmologists, is no longer used.

Vision therapy is a form of neurophysiologic treatment for a "disorder" or "dysfunction" and as such, does not usually treat disease. Specialists in brain function and behavioral therapy may be ideologically closer to developmental or behavioral optometrists than standard trained optometrists and ophthalmologists. Optometrists qualified to treat vision therapy as well as optometrists with dual degrees in psychology know how critical vision is to individual personality and how much vision can change personality and visa versa.

For all of these reasons, it may not be easy to find a qualified vision therapist in your neighborhood but whatever path is necessary to give you access to a vision therapy fellow is well worth the journey. A fellow is one who has taken and passed oral and written tests relating to vision therapy. Stories shared by patients who are products of vision therapy are both touching and relentless. Many patients are so compelled to tell the story of their successes and satisfaction that some become optometrists themselves, while others publish their own books to share their story with the public.

Sue Barry is one such patient. Dr. Barry is a neurobiologist and professor at Mount Holyoke College. She has been nicknamed "Stereo Sue" due to the visual problems experienced over a lifetime of only seeing in 2-D. Dr. Barry had little, if any, depth perception, but vision therapy changed that. After a lifetime of stereo blindness, Sue sought the expert care of a developmental optometrist and successfully completed optometric vision therapy. In 2006, Oliver Sacks discussed her story in *The New Yorker* (Sacks O 2006), as well as writing a chapter about her in 2010 in his book, *The Mind's Eye* (Sacks O 2010). In 2009 Sue published her own book, *Fixing My Gaze* (Barry 2009), based upon her positive experience with optometric vision therapy.

Many patients have published their own books while others have launched their own YouTube videos to publicly share their success with optometric vision therapy. Antonia Orfield, a patient turned behavioral optometrist published, *Eyes for Learning: Preventing and Curing Vision Related Learning Problems,* in 2007. Dr. Orfield found that remedies to vision related problems in children had a direct positive influence on test scores and grades and published her observations.

Not only did Dr. Orfield's own experience as a patient of optometric vision therapy lead her to become a behavioral optometrist but also she was motivated to open a vision clinic at the Mather Elementary School in Dorchester, MA in 1993. At that clinic, Dr. Orfield tested over 800 children and over 50% of the children failed the comprehensive vision examination. (www.visiontherapystories.org). Most of these students who failed had 20/20 eyesight, an evaluation that merely checks clarity of letters at a distance, but does not pick up visual problems or lack of fusion at a close range, the range required for reading.

When reading is difficult, kids just give up. Later many are mislabeled as learning disabled or as having an attention deficit disorder. (Eide and Eide 2006)

Finding the Right Kind of Help

When calling a developmental or behavioral eye doctor that involves a distance to drive, the following questions may prove helpful in locating a clinician who will meet your needs and make the commute a positive experience.

- The first question to ask is whether or not the office offers vision therapy. The answer should be affirmed with an additional response that reflects a strong level of enthusiasm for offering vision therapy.

- Is the vision therapy provided as "in-office" therapy or is it an "at-home" approach? Vision therapy should be provided on site in the office under appropriate professional supervision.

- How many vision therapy patients does the doctor see each week? Eye doctors who enthusiastically treat vision therapy patients generally invest additional professional continuing education time as well as invest in expanded equipment in the vision therapy learning labs in their offices. With such a high level of professional commitment, vision therapy becomes their specialty and soon more patients seek their services. This is usually indicative of an experienced vision therapy specialist.

- What professional organizations does the optometric vision therapist belong to and at what level is their membership? Are they certified at the fellowship level?

VISION THERAPY: THE BASICS

The retina divides the old from the new in the practice of professional eye care. This thin membrane at the back of the eyeball is where sight and vision meet. The retina is where light that has entered the eye at the cornea and been focused by the lens is transformed into electrical messages to be sent to the brain for interpretation.

Eye doctors who practice vision therapy are primarily concerned with what happens behind the retina, in the interaction between brain and eyes, *the world of vision.* Traditional eye care is limited to what happens in front of, and at, the retina, *the world of sight.* Its practitioners treat what are called "refractive errors," of which the most common are, as we have observed, myopia (nearsightedness), hyperopia (farsightedness) and astigmatism, all of which are due to an improperly shaped eyeball. The improper shape prevents the image focused by the lens from falling accurately on the retina. If the eyeball is elongated from front to back, the distance from lens to retina is too great, and the image focuses before the retina; the result is myopia. If the eyeball is too shallow, the focus falls, theoretically, beyond the retina, and that is farsightedness.

Astigmatism is due to an irregularly shaped eyeball that distorts the focus. Eyeglasses or contact lenses that compensate for the effects of the misshapen eyeball and cause the image to fall accurately on the retina readily treat all three. Such prescribing, plus in some cases medical or surgical treatment, is the self-imposed limit of traditional eye practice.

HOW THE EYE WORKS

Light enters the eye through the cornea, the fluid-filled bulge at the front of the eyeball. The cornea slows down the light and bends it toward the center. The light now reaches the iris, which narrows or expands the dark hole at its center, the pupil, to regulate the amount of light that proceeds toward the retina. The iris narrows in bright light, dilates when light is dim. This in turn changes the size of the pupil, which is actually a "hole" in the iris.

The lens focuses the light when the cilliary muscle changes its shape; this sharpens the picture the lens has received from the cornea. To reach the retina, the image now passes through the ball of clear jelly that makes up the greater part of the eye. This "vitreous humor" exerts fluid pressure that maintains the eyeball's shape. (Occasional vague shapes we see before our eyes are dead blood cells floating in the jelly.)

The retina is a thin membrane at the back of the eyeball. The macula, a small area near the center of the retina, is the region of greatest visual acuity. Sight is keenest of all at the fovea, the tiny pit at the center of the macula. When we turn our eyes toward what we want to look at, we are aligning them so that light falls directly on the fovea.

The retina is where the image, first recorded by the cornea and modified along the way, is translated into electrical messages carried by the optic nerves to those parts of the brain where we interpret what our eyes record.

Developmental or behavioral optometry, as the specialty is called, is concerned not just with how well people see but with how well they are able to use their eyes and how comfortably they can sustain visual concentration.

Good sight as designated by a score of 20/20 on the eye chart is not enough. Total functioning vision is better than "good eyesight" and many who pass the 20/20 test can fail a complete visual exam. When you have an eye exam you should expect to be evaluated for your ability to make full use of your vision. The purpose of vision therapy is to remedy visual disorders that prevent people from enjoying full use of vision. For example, the exam should show how both eyes work together and how visual information is processed and interpreted.

The symptoms of visual disorders show up in the eyes, but the causes lie elsewhere. This bears repeating: *symptoms of visual disorders show up in the eyes, but the causes lie elsewhere.* The problems are found in the interpretation by the brain of

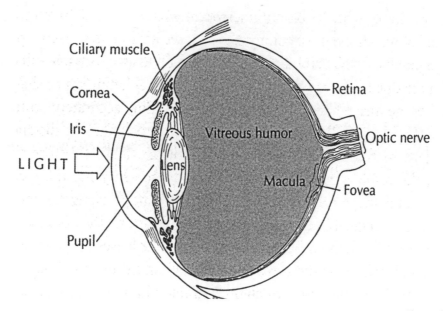

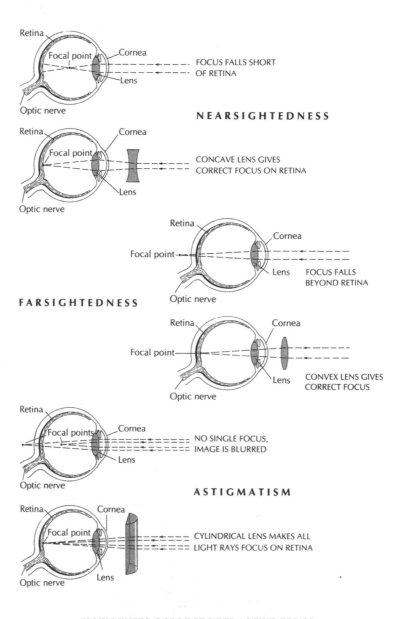

Retina
Focal point
Cornea
Lens
Optic nerve

FOCUS FALLS SHORT
OF RETINA

NEARSIGHTEDNESS

Retina
Focal point
Cornea
Lens
Optic nerve

CONCAVE LENS GIVES
CORRECT FOCUS ON RETINA

Retina
Focal point
Cornea
Lens
Optic nerve

FOCUS FALLS
BEYOND RETINA

FARSIGHTEDNESS

Retina
Focal point
Cornea
Lens
Optic nerve

CONVEX LENS GIVES
CORRECT FOCUS

Retina
Focal points
Cornea
Lens
Optic nerve

NO SINGLE FOCUS,
IMAGE IS BLURRED

ASTIGMATISM

Retina
Focal point
Cornea
Lens
Optic nerve

CYLINDRICAL LENS MAKES ALL
LIGHT RAYS FOCUS ON RETINA

HOW LENSES CORRECT REFRACTIVE ERROR.

the messages received from the eyes and in the instructions the brain then sends back to the eyes.

The most visible and familiar disorder of vision is known as strabismus, which means that one or both eyes are turned, sometimes up or down but usually in or out: the person is cross-eyed or walleyed. Amblyopia, or lazy eye, is a related problem but is less obvious than strabismus. One eye sees but does not function properly in conjunction with its partner, so the brain suppresses its messages and in effect gets along with the information supplied by the other eye.

Orthoptics, the precursor of today's vision therapy, had its origins in the treatment of strabismus in the late 19th century. The French ophthalmologist Emile Javal developed a series of training routines as an alternative to eye surgery after seeing the results of eye muscle surgery performed on both his father and his sister. He described the surgery he witnessed as "le massacre des muscles oculaires." Or "the massacre of the muscles of the eye."

Today some practitioners still treat strabismus with surgery though the success rate is significantly lower compared to success achieved by vision therapy. "Success" in this case means that the two eyes function effectively together. While surgery may correct the appearance of the eye, it does so without assuring good visual functioning. This makes the surgical solution to the problem a solution laden with high risk and a gamble for good outcomes at best.

Disorders of "binocular fusion" involve difficulties in using the eyes as a team. Binocular vision is a complex process involving several sets of nerves and muscles. All we are aware of is that with our conscious mind we tell our eyes to direct their attention to the so-called 'object of regard'. The response seems to us immediate but involves several successive actions ordered by the brain: it tells one set of muscles to turn the eyes in or out; instructs other muscles to bring the eyes together so that the image falls on the center of each retina, then to fuse the two images into one; and finally tells a muscle in each eyeball to adjust the lens to focus the image. A malfunctioning in any of these systems will make binocular vision difficult to achieve and especially difficult to sustain. Unlike crossed eyes or walleyes, these disorders are not immediately visible. They manifest themselves most often when a person has trouble with that most necessary and visually demanding tasks of modern life, reading, computer work and similar kinds of concentrated work. Reading with such a disorder will be uncomfortable and sometimes painful.

Since, as noted, the causes of all visual disorders lie in the messages sent by the eye to the brain, that is also where vision therapy takes place. Vision is learned, and in therapy the brain learns to do it better. Vision therapy trains the brain to give the correct instructions to the muscles of the eye. The instruments we use are designed to help create situations in which the brain finds it natural to give those correct instructions. In addition, vision therapy teaches the patient to process and interpret visual data more efficiently. This then affects conceptual skills as well as thinking skills.

Training routines are designed to isolate the different functions of binocular vision and work on those that need help. The routines typically consist of doing familiar tasks under unfamiliar conditions. The patient will read, or draw, or follow a moving object with his eyes. He may do so while looking through Polaroid glasses that separate the sight in the two eyes so that the brain cannot rely on one eye alone but must practice its use of the other, or through a prism that stimulates his ability to move his eyes in and out in tandem, or through lenses that alternately stimulate and relax the focusing system.

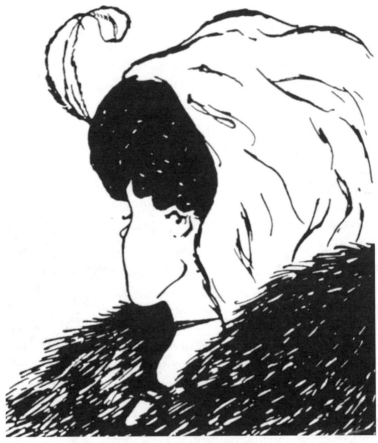

FIGURE VERSUS GROUND

In this drawing you see either an old woman or a young one. You can see them alternately, but you cannot see them both at the same time. This is how the brain achieves visual concentration. By organizing visual information to perceive one representation, the figure, it temporarily excludes competing information, the ground.

People who have difficulty with figure ground discrimination are likely to have trouble concentrating on written information. For example, a child looking at a page full of arithmetic problems may find it hard or impossible to concentrate visually on one problem to the exclusion of the others. Then, by definition, a person with figure ground deficiencies will have difficulty attending and concentrating on visual information. Psychologist E.G. Boring devised this picture and is known as "Wife/mistress."

With enough practice, the brain learns to send the right instructions to the eyes without the help of the therapist's devices. Once a person reaches this point, the cure usually is lasting, for then the habit of doing it right is reinforced during every waking moment; it becomes easier and more comfortable to do it right. It is not like a workout that must be repeated daily to keep the muscles in shape.

Choosing An Eye Doctor

Today many eye doctors who offer vision therapy are optometrists certified by the College of Optometrists in Vision Development (COVD). To find an eye doctor who offers vision therapy, ask your family eye doctor to refer you or search the following websites: www.oepf.org; www.helpaddvisiontherapy.com; www.COVD.org.

Other kinds of visual and vision related skills could be improved with vision therapy. Skills such as peripheral vision and visual reaction time, essential in driving and for many sports, can readily be developed with practice on therapeutic instruments. The same is true for perceptual skills, which are often undeveloped in children who experience learning difficulties in the early years of school. Examples are eye-hand coordination, visual memory, and figure-ground perception, which is the ability to separate the essential from the irrelevant in what one sees.

For some, "vision therapy" may call up the image of eye exercises, which implies that therapy somehow strengthens our eyes. Conceptualizing vision therapy as exercise is misleading. (Today's vision therapy should not be confused with the routines prescribed by the "Bates method" that was popular several decades ago.)

Eye muscles are anywhere from 50 to 100 times stronger than they need to be to do the work we ask of them. What is accomplished by vision therapy might better be compared to learning to type on a keyboard, playing the piano or learning to ride a bicycle. For all of these learned activities it is not the strength of the muscles that matters but rather the ability the muscles possess.

What can we do with our muscles and how do we signal muscles to perform is what is at the heart of the matter. Learning muscle function skill is to teach the brain to send the correct message to the body for a specific outcome. Vision therapy trains the brain to send correct signals to and from the eyes and body. This all takes practice, not muscle development. The therapist must know where the patient is at in their stage of development, where they need to go and what further development needs to happen. Then a program is designed in which the patient succeeds at a rate of at least 85% to 95% level. The demands are increased until the desired level of performance is achieved.

As one might suppose, the likely duration and chance of success in vision therapy depends mainly on the nature of the problem and the state of the patient. A young, healthy, motivated person with a disorder that is not too severe has an excellent chance of a quick, complete, and lasting cure. With more complicated patients, therapy may take longer and involve more effort with an equally as successful outcome. Vision therapy, when managed by an experienced practitioner, has a track record for 90% success rate in treating the most common visual disorders. In general, a course of vision therapy typically involves an hour or two per week

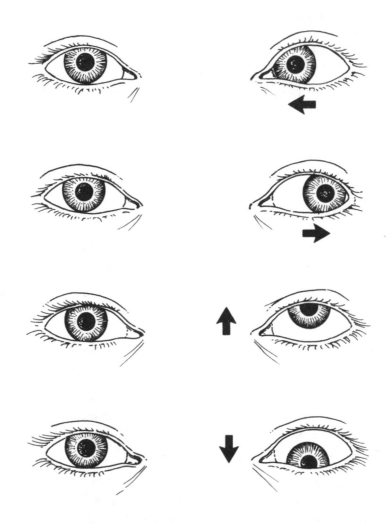

TYPES OF STRABISMUS

and usually takes between three to nine months to complete. However, the patient usually reports noticing changes after only a few sessions.

Successful therapy is measured in two ways. The patient judges one way. Are they performing better and feeling better? Did the therapy solve the initial problems that brought them in for help? The second way is by the eye doctor who is able to objectively measure improvement and continually monitor clinical accuracy. Each visual skill is measured before and after treatment with diagnostic tests that yield objective results. As one would expect, the results of these tests are typically echoed by the patient's own observations of their own improvement.

In the chapters that follow, we describe the role that vision therapy plays in people's lives from childhood to retirement, in activities as diverse as working at a video display terminal, rehabilitating juvenile delinquents, reading comprehension, attention span and concentration, as well as driving with increased safety.

Meanwhile, the contribution that vision therapy has made to the competitive athlete is a topic unto itself. Extreme visual acuity and extreme improvements in visual reaction time, visualization, visual tracking and perceptual awareness, that trained professional athletes have exhibited have both surprised and even surpassed what vision therapists themselves would envision what therapy could do. It is all possible to learn to do.

References

Barry SR 2009. Fixing My Gaze: A Scientist's Journey into Seeing in three Dimensions. New York: Basic Books.

Eide B, Eide F 2006. The Mislabeled Child: Looking Beyond Behavior to Find the True Sources and Solutions for Children's Learning Challenges. New York: Hyperion.

Orfield A 2007. Eyes for Learning: Preventing and Curing Vision-Related Learning Problems. Blue Ridge Summit, PA: Rowman & Littlefield Education.

Sacks O 2006. A Neurologist's Notebook: "Stereo Sue." The New Yorker. June 19, 2006:64.

Sacks O 2010 2009. The Mind's Eye. New York: Alfred A. Knopf.

Recommended Reading

Duckman R. Visual Development, Diagnosis and Treatment of the Pediatric Patient. Philadelphia: Lippincott, Williams and Wilkins, 2006.

Orfield A 1994. Seeing Space: Undergoing Brain Reprogramming to Reduce Myopia. Journal of Behavioral Optometry 5:123–31.

Orfield A, Basa F, Yun J 2001. Vision problems of children in poverty in an urban school clinic: heir epidemic numbers, impact on learning, and approaches to remediation. Journal of Optometric Vision Development 32: 114–141.

CHAPTER 3
HOW VISION DEVELOPS:
THE PRESCHOOL YEARS

"The most pathetic person in the world is someone who has sight but no vision." Helen Keller 1880-1968

Let's begin with Piaget. Jean Piaget was an epistemologist known for his work on how thinking evolves. Simply put, he was curious about how children during their development, come to know what they know. Fascinated by his own three children, Jacqueline, Lucienne and Laurent, he based his theories on his intense observation of them. According to Piaget, children's cognitive development falls into four stages that relate to skill, children's ways of understanding and interpreting the world around them.

The first stage is the sensorimotor stage. It occurs from birth to two years. At this age children enjoy touching, holding, and looking at objects. Most of what they relate to in the world is through their senses. This is why children at this age are fascinated with mobiles above their crib, sounds from rattles, and grabbing a fuzzy stuffed toy. Around 9 months of age they begin to sense permanence in the world. Permanence is often reflected in the game children play "peek-a-boo." When the child covers his eyes, he or she thinks that since he can't see you that you can't see him. At this stage, children also love toys that require them to see, listen, touch and hide.

The second, or "pre-operational" stage of development, according to Piaget, is between the ages 2 years and 7 years. At this time children begin to think and communicate in symbols. Now letters, numbers and words start to gain meaning. This stage is very important because this is when children start to develop a concept of a self. The ability to organize and plan ahead, or set goals and achieve them is developed during this time, too. To be able to start and finish things as well as concentrate on the process to do so is critically woven into this phase.

The primary characteristic of the second stage is that the child is dominated by his or her visual perceptions. At this stage, children make a wonderful audience for a magician because they believe everything they see. If they have a choice between a *big* chocolate bar or a *small* bag of m&ms® (both of equal weight), they'll choose the bag of m&m's® because it looks like more because it has multiple pieces. In addition, the different colors of the m&m's® make the choice spectacular.

This is also the time when children develop the ability to "regulate" their actions. For example, not to disrupt other students, not to do or say inappropriate things and to be able to discern right and wrong behavior. Today, these skills may also be referred to as "executive function skills." (Wecker, Kramer, Wisniewski, Delis and Kaplan 2000)

As children approach 7 years of age and move on to the next phase called the concrete operations phase, they start to develop skills to plan ahead and conserve resources. Learning to read, to recognize symbols, letters, and numbers and understand cause effect relationships, all develop in this stage, which usually continues through approximately age 11. During this stage, thought patterns are concrete. Ideas are based upon things they directly observe and thinking is "black and white" so to speak.

Once children are around age 11, they begin to develop abstract reasoning skills. Teaching youngsters in this age group requires demonstration, hands-on activities and experimentation in science class. Kids this age benefit from an educational environment that has clear objectives and requires them to combine ideas and think critically. This stage is called the state of formal operations stage and usually begins around age 12. It should be noted that there is a surprising percentage of children who do not reach this stage, even by the time they are 17 years old. This raises all sorts of questions. Imagine that group of teenagers who do not reach this level of development. How do teachers and schools handle this developmental gap in the classroom? Hold back the students who are right on track? Ignore the needs of the lesser developed students? Do they label these kids as "learning disabled" or consider them as having ADD/ADHD and recommend drugs to stabilize the classroom?

Teaching strategies for this stage of development should require a higher order of information processing and expect students to interpret, defend, combine, explain, debate, hypothesize and construct ideas. Mostly, this should be the stage where they learn to understand someone else's viewpoint.

For Piaget, each of these stages builds upon the previous phase, and are not fully realized if one of the stages is compromised. Since vision is considered to be 80% of a child's experience with the world during all phases, visual ability and potential cannot be over emphasized here. Visual perception and visual perceptual motor skills are critical during the second phase in particular and the transition to the third stage. This stage in particular, when a child's "self identity" is developing is also the time when reading begins. This is also when a child should start to become "attached" or grounded in their environment.

When attachment is compromised, when kids do not fully develop a self identity, and when they seem scattered as opposed to grounded in their everyday behavior, they are sitting ducks for a wide range of future problems. Some kids may withdraw while others 'act out.' Some may appear hyperactive, while others appear depressed and mope. At the extreme end some may develop pervasive developmental disorders such as Asperger's or autism, while others are attracted to drugs.

For more information on ADD, ADHD vs. CI (convergence insufficiency disorder) in vision, please see Chapter 5. In addition there are numerous educational handbooks on Piaget's work for teachers and parents. Please see the reference list at the end of this chapter for further reading, particularly the books recommended for teachers and parents.

This chapter is on early child development, but you can see how early child development lays the groundwork for what will follow. Let's turn again to the needs of early childhood as it relates to vision. Drug addiction, ADD, ADHD, Asperger's and autism are covered in chapters that follow. We start life with the potential for vision, but vision itself is acquired through our own efforts since vision is a learned activity. How well we succeed in those efforts goes a long way toward determining how well we will function in the world.

Summarizing the thoughts of physician Arnold Gesell, pioneer in the study of children's vision, children are "born with a pair of eyes, but not with a visual world. They must build that world by themselves, and it is their own private creation. The space world thus becomes part of each child. To no small degree, each child is part of it." In humans the development of vision is relatively slow. A chick has vision virtually from the moment of birth, on its first day after hatching. It shows in that it can coordinate eye and bill, successfully pecking its food. For people, by contrast, it takes about 10 years, often more, for the visual system to achieve complete development, and even then it is continually developing and forever changing.

Vision develops not by itself but in intimate relation with the growth of our other abilities, such as the use of our bodies and minds. Each stage of physical and mental development has its visual aspect, and understanding that visual aspect is essential to understanding the child's growth. The development of vision, however, is far less conspicuous than the stages of other kinds of growth. We can easily observe a child learning to crawl, to walk, to talk, but we cannot as easily see the subtle visual learning that accompanies each of those advances. We can tell at a glance that a 5 year old is not fully grown, but that glance does not tell us if his or her visual system is ready for the demands of school. Understanding of the role of vision has crucial implications for the care of children.

The world to a newborn is small, and so too is their visual world. Newborn babies see no farther than about 8 inches, which is the distance to their mother's face. At that age, babies cannot coordinate their eyes, and they usually appear to be staring rather than looking, and perception, for the most part, comes through the sense of touch, taste and hearing.

What happens, starting at birth, can best be described as reaching out to grasp the world, first with the hands, then with the eyes, which extend the child's grasp beyond the reach of the arms and other senses. As the visual grasp increases, babies come to rely more and more on vision for information. This is an amazing process which enables babies to develop basic survival skills that develop the use of vision to capture and understand the world in which they must function in order to survive. These are not smooth advances, but rather spurts of growth periods followed by rest periods that allow the child to process and master the space just added to their own private visual world. That world is what Richard S. Kavner (1985), in his excellent book, *Your Child's Vision*, calls the child's "personal space."

By the time a baby is 6 months old, they have begun to coordinate their eyes with their arm movements, and are able to shift attention. Shifts in attention are necessary for eye-hand coordination, an important forerunner for that skill. By 6 months of age a baby is starting to learn to focus on objects at close range. This is the beginning of the long process of developing binocular vision, the use of the eyes as a team, that enables us to understand and measure space.

Binocular vision enables each eye to coordinate with the other, blending two separate images into one providing better close range vision as well as depth perception. In order to better understand how the brain plays a role in binocular vision, it may be helpful to think of animals that do and don't have the same type of vision as humans. Take for example, rabbits or horses, or any animal that has eyes located on opposite sides of the head. This type of vision gives the widest possible view, but with less depth and precision. Animals with eyes positioned on opposite sides of the head need to protect themselves from predators and need a wider field of vision than humans need. Predatory animals as well as birds can have up to a 360° range of vision because each eye has the ability to move independently up down and sideways.

Humans, however, as well as wolves, eagles and other animals that need to master specific skills at close range as well as have visual acuity, have forward facing eyes. Forward facing eyes reduce the field of peripheral vision but increase depth perception and visual precision at close range. When we speak of close range vision, we are referring to a whole group of processed skills in the range of an arm's length. Each example of an animal, bird or mammal that has eyes closer to the front of the face requires an increase in the way the brain interprets and interacts with visual input and eye motor output.

With binocular vision the eyes coordinate and move together. When we are born we see with the left eye as well as the right eye. The brain must go through the process of learning to eliminate the double images received by eyes that are not yet quite coordinated and not yet working together.

To think of binocular vision as anything less than a complex process of eye-brain coordination is to view the world of human vision as that of a Cyclops. The process of brain-eye training is complex, and as a result some children learn faster while others compensate by having the non-dominant eye shut down.

When the field of view of the left eye overlaps with the field of the right eye, and does not fuse both images into one, the brain gets confused. The brain receives more than one image of the same object, and vision is double. The brain compensates for the confusion by ignoring some of the information it receives. The brain then suppresses or turns off the image from one eye. If the brain does not suppress the second image, the result is double vision. The brain's suppression of select images also explains why some people experience words that jump or disappear on a page, and why some people reverse letters or word order.

If the brain doesn't selectively ignore overlapping input from individual eyes, the person who actually has double vision gets by in the world by falling into one of three unconscious categories. This is the body's way of solving the problem within itself.

AVOIDANCE

The first manner in which the brain deals with binocular visual dysfunctions (double vision) is to inadvertently avoid engaging in tasks that require visual concentration at close range. In this way, they only have to deal with visual activities that require focusing at a distance beyond the field of double vision.

Visual activity avoidance solves a whole range of problems for the brain, but with that, comes an aversion to reading. People whose brains have chosen this route to solve the double vision dilemma usually do not read well, and when they do comprehension is compromised. They are also slow readers, and easily fall behind in all respects. As you can well imagine, with this category of unconscious binocular defect management, a person may have a high IQ, yet read, test and perform at a level significantly below their intellectual potential. On top of that, they may also be inattentive or hyperactive in situations that require close concentration or lengthy reading. Many people exhibiting these traits are also mislabeled as ADD or ADHD. Once again, it is important to have accurate follow-up by a qualified vision therapist with any type of casual diagnosis.

MENTAL MOTIVATION

The second way in which the brain manages the dilemma of double vision is through mental motivation. Some people are determined to succeed at any cost. They endure headaches while reading, deal with continual frustration, manage chronic discomfort, tire easily and are willing to pay the continual price for the consequences they feel from engaging in close work. People in this category often are agitated, angry and even difficult to deal with because they experience chronic low-grade pain on a daily basis. They may even be misdiagnosed as having migraines, depression, attention spectrum disorders, and may even be driven to addictive substances to endure the continual mental and physical pain.

SUPPRESSION

The brain learns to suppress the image from one eye.

The link between myopia and close work activities has been scientifically documented. (White, 2001) In this study, it was determined that high achieving students, as well as highly educated adults in general, who engage in work at close range (reading, studying, computer work and graphic design) tend to have increased incidents of myopia. Myopic vision disorder has increased in developed countries over the last 100 years. This particular study, conducted in Singapore, revealed close to a 400% increase in myopia among students in academically accelerated programs. Similar increases have been documented in students completing intense precollege courses. As illustrated in Chapter One, the Snellen Test identifies people in the third category, but only by identifying the symptoms and measuring the consequences of double vision. The Snellen Test does not identify double vision, but may be a good measure of its consequences.

Failure to pass the Snellen Test should signal the next aspect of the eye exam to include a visual examination for double vision. To diagnose myopia and stop at the Snellen Test results is to be incomplete in assessing total vision. The diagnosis of myopia should include a complete assessment of total vision and the brain's relationship to the eyes along with the dispensing of the prescription for corrective lenses. Anything less than a complete visual exam for the myopic patient is nothing short of supervised neglect.

This is one of many examples of a disorder of binocular vision that can be helped with vision therapy. Vision therapy helps teach the brain to eliminate double vision, not by ignoring input to the brain, but by teaching the brain to fuse the images. In this way, double vision is eliminated by correcting it rather than by selectively ignoring information.

By the age of 6 months, infants have very little depth perception. Their personal space now extends to around 2 feet, give or take the individual child. Some children will progress slower with no cause for alarm unless they fall far behind the norm. Between 8 and 12 months the child's personal space extends to around 3 feet, well beyond the reach of their hands. Their eyes focus well in that near space, and they now notice objects in a mid-range of 3 to 10 feet. Children this age can recognize their mother's face, which is a complex achievement of vision and brain activity. This means that he or she have begun to have visual memory: the ability to store an image in the mind. They can now scan an object, mother's face for example, with the eyes and separate out the details they need from all other information the eyes are sending. From the visual memory they can now compare the resulting shape with the image in their memory and conclude that the pictures match. They can identify that the person they are looking at is their mother.

By age 2, a child must learn to use vision in correlation with rapidly expanding bodily abilities. Two year olds need vision to help them walk and talk. As they learn to talk, children make another complex advance in the use of vision and mind. The child begins to integrate vision with language, thus what they see begins to relate to language, heard and spoken. This skill will be the bedrock of academic learning that will occupy many of the years to come. Mastery of audio-visual skills is as necessary to the survival of a young child today growing up in the age of technology as it was to the development of the hunting skills of his ancestors. By the time a child is 2 years old we can notice that their eyes are beginning to lead their actions. Vision, the sense with the longest reach and the only sense that can scan, is starting to take over as the primary tool of perception. At this age, children can turn head and eyes without turning the body. They can see another person's eyes 5 to 8 feet away, and binocular vision extends to between 2 and 3 feet. Even though they have binocular vision, it is far from perfect in the 2 to 3 foot range of space.

At 2 years of age, the absence of binocular vision is not always easy to pick up. At times the eyes visibly drift apart, but at other times the child's eyes may be moving as a team. They appear to be focusing on the object of interest while the brain may not yet have achieved the ability to fuse the two images enabling space to be seen in three dimensions.

Around 2 years of age, children achieve yet another complex advance. They begin, just begin, to visualize a hypothetical action. At this stage of development children begin to see in the mind's eye what would happen if they were to put this object in that place. They can visually imagine a toy falling off the edge of a table, instead of having to find out by trial and error as he or she did before they acquired visual intuition. By the age of 2, the child is beginning to understand the concept of cause and effect; another way that vision and mind develop in tandem.

By now, 2 year olds are also sensing that the world is a permanent place. The visual aspect of permanence dissipates the infantile feeling that the world disappears when the eyes are covered or closed. Before permanence, the games of hide and seek involved covering the eyes to make the world disappear. After acquiring the sense of permanence, children know that the world doesn't work that way. At this time, they also do better at coordinating the senses, turning the head, for example, to see what they just heard.

By about halfway through the third year after birth, children start to show verbal understanding of the space they are mastering with vision. Concepts behind such words as "near," "far," "up," "down," "on" and "under" are solidifying. But the visual world is still precarious, and a 3 year old is still largely dependent on manual contact to understand the reality of their surroundings. If they lose touch of an object, they are likely to lose sight of it as well. Although 3 year olds are binocular in their near space, they cannot always coordinate their eyes, and one eye or the other may be seen to drift.

Three is a relatively stable age. Eye-hand movements are advanced enough so that, while drawing or painting, the child can keep the lines within the bounds of the paper. They can scan without moving the head, a skill important later on, and they can use their hands for one task while they direct their eyes elsewhere. Within the 3 year old's personal space, which now extends out to 7 to 10 feet, he or she is fully binocular.

At about 3 1/2 the child typically experiences a period of confusion during which they seem to regress. They sometimes stutter, stumble, or just simply fatigue. Newly acquired coordination skills between visual and motor systems are still immature. Between 3 and 4 years of age the visual world is uncertain because the child begins to explore space in new and different ways. Eye-hand movements and binocular vision may seem to work less well than when they were under 3 years old.

Age 4 is once again a stable period. The child can now maintain eye contact and concentrate their visual attention on distances of about 10 to 16 feet. This is close to the distance vision required to go to school when they are 5 years old. Four year olds can coordinate body and vision to catch and throw a ball, as well as follow the ball while it is in the air. At this age they are able to charge after the moving ball with smoothness during changing speeds.

Parents will, of course, want to provide the best conditions for their child's visual development. Along with the general principles of child rearing, two points are of particular importance. Children's vision needs to be stimulated. Since visual growth is a constant dynamic process of reaching out, it is important to provide the child with interesting things to look at that will draw attention beyond the present range of his or her vision.

It is equally important not to constrict the child's field of vision so they don't have a reason to expand beyond its reach. A perfect example is the visual aspect of the playpen, which limits the visual field of distance to a couple of feet. Leaving a child too often for too many hours in a playpen can discourage visual growth. In fact, the less time spent in the playpen, the better.

Outdoor play has the opposite effect. Indoor activities involve walls that define the distance of the of the child's visual field. When people of all ages are outdoors, they can gaze off as far as the horizon. "Go out and get some fresh air," parents will say. They might also say, at least to themselves: "Go outside and stretch your vision." One final concern regarding the development of vision from infancy through adulthood involves adherence to good nutrition. A well balanced diet with appropriate vitamin and mineral supplements is critical to, not only good vision, but to the health of the eyes as well as the brain.

Most people are already aware that including more fresh fruits and vegetables in the diet, as well as avoiding highly processed foods while also eliminating excess sugar, is just simple good common sense. In addition to this, many parents are also skeptical of food additives along with growth hormones, environmental estrogens, and pesticide residues that find their way into their child's system.

For parents interested in more detail on diet, food additives and family nutrition than is included in this chapter, additional information can be found online as well as in other published work. Briefly, the summary that follows, illustrates basic nutritional guidelines for healthy vision development.

Nutrition For Children's Vision

Balanced nutrition plays a central role in the development of a child's vision. Keep in mind that vitamin and mineral supplements are not regulated in the same way that prescription drugs are regulated, although they can be equally as influential in doing good, or causing harm to the body. The rule of thumb is to use supplements, in moderation, where a diet may be lacking. If you use dietary supplements, be sure to purchase them from reputable suppliers. In general, manufacturers who display the USP seal of approval are put through more rigorous testing, and are reliable sources.

A healthy amount of vitamin A is essential for healthy rods and cones in the retina, but it is important to avoid overdoses of this fat-soluble vitamin. Signs of deficiency include difficulty adjusting to darkness and changing intensities of light, a dry lusterless appearance of the cornea and surface of the eyeball, sties, burning or inflamed or itching eyes.

The B vitamins are also critical to good vision and a young child's vision development. Signs of deficiency include unclear vision, inflammation of internal eye tissues or ocular nerves, dry, burning sensation in the eye, double vision, weakening of the ocular muscles, involuntary oscillation of the eyeball, referred to as nystagmus.

Vitamin C, one of the most important antioxidants for the eye, is equally as important as vitamins A and B. Signs of vitamin C deficiency include sudden appearance of bulging of the eyes, known as exophthalmoses.

Calcium deficiencies can increase the severity of myopia and implicates Vitamin D, which, related to calcium absorption is important to good vision too. Studies reveal that Vitamin D deficiencies are on the rise. The nutrient chromium is also important in minimizing the risk of myopia as well as other problems with focusing.

Eye Chart For Preschool Children

Habitual squinting is the surest sign of nearsightedness. Parents noticing this behavior should seek out a complete visual exam for their child even if they seem too young for corrective lenses.

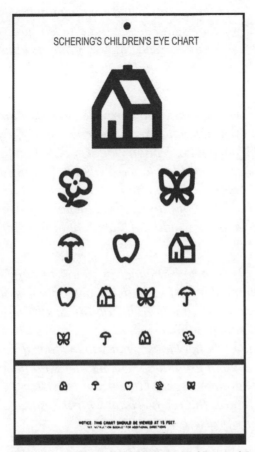

Reproduced by permission from Harold S. Stein, and Bernard J. Slatt and Raymond M. Stein: The Ophthalmic Assistant, 5th ed. (St. Louis:C.V. Mosby, 1988)

The literal meaning of the term "myopia" is "shut eye." The myopic child tends to be passive, to avoid much physical activity, and may shun risk. Because visual reach is limited, this type of child lives in a constricted world, preferring close-up sedentary activities. They often get very close to what they are doing, even burying their nose in their book. Michael B is one example of this type of child.

Michael *was 2 years old when his parents began to notice that something was wrong with his sight. Until then this unusually bright child had concealed his exceptionally poor sight. He rarely wanted to watch television, even avoiding "Sesame Street," and when he did watch, he would put his face almost up against the screen. One day while the family was looking at photos Michael brought each picture right up against his eyes. His parents decided they had to seek help. Two ophthalmologists who examined him said he was severely nearsighted and proposed only to fit him with full-strength glasses. Dissatisfied, the parents came to our office at the recommendation of one of our patients.*

Michael was about 2 1/2 when he started treatment with us. He was indeed severely myopic, one of that small percentage of children born very near-sighted. His blurred sight, we were certain, was going to cause him to miss out on the normal development of binocular vision. We believed he was headed for serious trouble when he got to school.

We started Michael with glasses that provided a less-than-full correction. Very myopic people often cannot take full correction at first, but must work up to it in stages. The partial correction would enable him to see well enough to develop his vision but would also keep his eyes trying to see better. We gradually increased his prescription–though never to full correction–so that by school age he would be able to see the blackboard. We changed him to contact lenses at age 4 so he would not start school wearing glasses. He has used contacts since then.

When he was 4 we also started Michael in vision therapy designed to help him develop both binocular vision and his perceptual skills. We aimed at improving his eye-hand coordination, his ability to distinguish objects visu-ally and his visual memory. Soon he would need those skills in school, and we wanted him to be ready. Michael took readily to the therapy, which lasted nine months. His parents were a great help. His mother said he felt when going to therapy that he was "going to school like his older sisters." The drawings he brought home went up on the refrigerator with the other children's school-work and were equally praised.

Michael, however, continued to struggle in spite of his motivation. At age 7, he returned for more therapy and it was obvious that his depth perception was not developing normally. At 9, Michael is doing very well in fourth grade. His mother reports that he is "an excellent student, in all the top groups." He is also an avid young athlete whose sports include some that are visually very demanding: he plays catcher in baseball, and plays tennis and basketball as well. (We have, however, asked his parents to keep him out of contact sports like football and even soccer, for fear of damage to his fragile retinas which, being very myopic, may be prone to detaching.) After school he likes to get out on his roller skates.

Although he is still very myopic, Michael's personality is not that of the, shy, studious, very nearsighted person. He is an exceptionally friendly, active, and outgoing child. His mother believes, as we do, that he would not have turned out this way had he started school wearing thick glasses, and handicapped by poor visual skills.

It is important to note that, though he has made enormous gains, Michael B is not yet out of the woods. At 9, he is entering the years in which so many people become progressively more nearsighted. But now, thanks to a new form of therapy, there is an excellent chance that Michael, with the use of advanced session therapy techniques, can be kept from becoming any more nearsighted than he is today.

STRABISMUS

Strabismus, a turned eye, is the most obvious of visual problems in a child or adult. Where other disorders can be observed only through their consequences, a turned eye is immediately noticeable. Usually the eye is turned in (crossed) or out (wall-eyed), but sometimes it is up or down. Since at age 3 or 4 a child's visual system is still unstable, it is normal for an eye to drift in or out occasionally, and parents should not overreact to a passing phenomenon. But if the eye is persistently turned for days on end in the same direction, the child's vision should be examined, and if that examination confirms the presence of strabismus, it is important to take prompt action to prevent lasting damage.

Strabismus usually shows up between the ages of 18 months and 5 years. It afflicts from 2 to 4% of the population. Each year about one million children show evidence of strabismus. Its causes are not fully understood. Sometimes a childhood illness such as chickenpox or an emotional trauma such as the death of a parent can produce strabismus by disrupting the ability of the two eyes to work together.

The consequences of strabismus go beyond the aesthetic. The preschool years, as we have seen, are when the child's mind devotes itself to learning the difficult skill of binocular vision. If one eye is turned, binocular vision is impossible because the brain is getting different images from the two eyes. Finding this intolerable, the brain simply rejects the messages sent by the turned eye and in effect sees with the one straight eye. In time, the ability to see in the turned eye fades with disuse and may disappear permanently. Strabismus in those early years may prevent the essential learning of binocular vision even if the affliction eventually disappears or is successfully treated later on. This is because the brain tends to learn visual skills at the usual time or not at all. So, in later years the growing child's mind will direct its attention elsewhere even if it has not mastered binocular vision.

Parents of a child with strabismus face three choices: doing nothing, surgery, and/ or vision therapy. (There is also a form of treatment using drugs that is seldom practiced today.)

Doing nothing is often advocated on the grounds that the child may outgrow his strabismus, and his turned eye will right itself without intervention. In our opinion this is a dangerous route to follow. It is quite true that the child may outgrow the visible cosmetic problem in the sense that the eyes will appear to be correctly aligned, but if he has missed the time for learning binocular vision, those two eyes will not actually be working together, and he will not perceive space in depth, which becomes a severe handicap. This child may also miss out on other forms of learning that depend on good visual development.

The same hazard applies to surgery. Surgeons will attempt to realign the eye by changing the balance of the eye muscles, though in many cases the eye muscles are in fact not imbalanced. This surgery may correct the cosmetic problem, but, as in the case of doing nothing, the child may be left without binocular vision. Often surgery does not even correct the cosmetic problem. The eye remains turned, or, sometimes after an interval of months or years, the eye will turn in a different direction. Nothing has been solved and the eye's capacity for recovery has been permanently weakened. The chance of success in surgical treatment of strabismus is about 20%, dismal odds for an action whose consequences are irreversible. All too often Emile Javal's description of such surgery as "the massacre of the ocular muscles" is as valid today as when this first practitioner of vision therapy wrote it a century and a half ago.

Vision therapy is the parents' third option. Unlike surgery, it has no irreversible consequences. If it fails to cure the strabismus, no damage has been done to the child's eye. Most of the time, however, vision therapy does not fail. Its success rate is about 75%, almost four times that of surgery. Early treatment, again, is important to increase the chances for natural learning of binocular vision and to head off the possible side effects of failure in the child's first experiences in school.

> **Jessica** *was 4 1/2 when her parents began to notice something was wrong. Her right eye turned in and stayed that way, not like the wandering eye common in young children. She turned her head to look at people. She was unusually clumsy. Repeatedly she would trip over things she should have seen. She fell down much too often. Worried about kindergarten, which Jessica was about to enter, her parents brought her to us. Jessica suffered from alternating strabismus. Each eye would turn in separately from time to time. The brain finds it difficult to cope with the garbled messages sent by the eyes. When Jessica turned her head, it was an attempt to avoid seeing double. She was half a year behind in the development of her perceptual skills.*

> *We started Jessica on a course of vision therapy, combined with home exercises, which lasted nine months. For the first three months we asked Jessica to wear an eye patch over her better left eye during therapy to help induce her turned right eye to work. She took to the therapy readily, both in our office and at home. According to her parents, "It was something of her own."*

> *Jessica's therapy started just before her year in kindergarten. At first she could not see the blackboard except from the front row, and she had trouble drawing pictures and forming letters. By the end of the school year her scholastic problems had vanished. She could see the board, and her visual skills were up to normal. Her parents reported that she was "enthusiastic about reading."*

> *In her perceptual skills, Jessica had taken a remarkable leap forward, from half a year behind average to four years and eight months above average, all*

in nine months. Therapy had brought about this sudden great advance in two ways. First, it enabled her to use skills she already had, and second, it added to those skills. Jessica no longer fell down more than other children her age. She could now catch a playground ball which she could not do earlier in the year.

Jessica's once-turned eyes were now normal both in appearance and in function. The cosmetic problem was gone and so was the visual problem. Jessica's strabismus was completely cured—without surgery.

Perceptual problems usually manifest themselves in the child's motor skills because the eyes lead the physical actions—a mistaken lead causes a mistaken action. If the child is lagging in the growth of his motor skills and no pathology is present, it is likely to be because of a visual problem. Any such lag should flash a warning signal; this child may have a learning problem when enrolled in school. If lagging in several skills, the possibility becomes a probability. Similarly, a child who has worn an orthopedic brace is more likely to have a visual motor problem in school since motor impediment will have affected visual learning as well.

Parents should watch for any difficulty the child might have in successive motor milestones such as sitting up, crawling, creeping and walking. Other symptoms to watch for are dragging one leg; putting shoes on the wrong foot, trouble learning to tie laces or button, and unusual clumsiness. A child with a perceptual-motor problem is likely to have trouble learning to skip, and on stairs (especially going down) may tend to go one step at a time. This may also be suggestive of difficulty with bilateral interweaving. These children may also avoid doing puzzles.

Keep in mind that children must crawl before they can walk, and must pass through each of the motor milestones if their skills are to develop properly. Parents should not attempt to bypass a skill with which the child is having trouble, but rather help them master it. For many of the motor skills, there are games on the market that can enhance a child's opportunity to learn. Parents may also take the child to a developmental/behavioral optometrist to see if there is a visual perceptual problem that can be treated.

*When she was very young, **Lindsay**'s parents observed that something was wrong. Although she was a bright, alert child, she kept bumping into things. She complained frequently of headaches, and she was afraid to go to bed because of the shadows she thought she was seeing. Two eye practitioners found nothing wrong with Lindsay's sight, but a third, a specialist in vision therapy, diagnosed amblyopia, or lazy eye.*

Lindsay was getting virtually no information from her left eye—only shadows—although there appeared to be nothing wrong with the eye itself. The cause in her case, was what is called anisometropia. The sight in the two eyes is so different that the brain is unable, even with glasses, to reconcile the conflicting images it is receiving, suppresses the messages from one eye. Lindsay was extremely farsighted in one eye, hardly at all in the other.

The eye doctor prescribed a patch for her good right eye which would force the lazy left eye to do its share of the work. Lindsay, then 4, wore the patch for three months, and the treatment was successful. Lindsay's headaches vanished and so did the frightening shadows. She went off to school and did well in the first three grades. She learned to read on schedule and did well in sports.

In fourth grade the required reading increased the demands on her vision to the point where she once again needed therapy. But the patch had given her crucial help in the all important first years of school, a high payoff for a simple noninvasive form of therapy.

At about age 5 the child will enter school. Now for the first time he will have to keep pace with others. He will have to perform to standards set not by his own rate of maturing but by the teacher and the other members of the group. A delay of six months in his visual development, which might otherwise be harmless, can have damaging effects in school by impeding his performance. If he is failing in his first experience in this new environment, the child is likely to be soured on school and to turn against learning in general.

Just as the body is not fully grown, at 5 a child's visual system is still not fully developed. It will go on developing for another five years or longer, though the rate of change will slow down. By age five the child's vision needs to demonstrate certain well defined levels if he or she is to meet the expectations of school.

His most obvious need is for visual acuity in order to see what the teacher is doing at the front of the room. The Snellen wall chart with its big E, and the expression of normal sight as 20/20, are based on the assumption that the child needs normal sight at 20 feet, which was taken to be the average distance to the blackboard. 20/20 means that one sees at 20 feet what the normal eye sees at that distance. 20/40 means that one sees at 20 feet what the normal eye sees at 40 feet. 20/10 means one sees at 20 feet what the normal eye sees at 10 feet. Acuity as measured by the Snellen or a similar chart is a function of the size and shape of the eyeball, not a skill the child has learned. Acuity is also the only aspect of a child's sight that is routinely examined when starting school.

The child needs another set of visual skills, not measured by the Snellen chart, that differ from acuity in two essential ways. They are learned skills, and they involve movement. Any deficiency is due to a delay in learning, not to a flaw in the eyeball to be corrected by glasses. Though the child will continue to improve these skills for the next five years or more, he must have reached certain minimum levels by the time he starts school in order to cope with its demands. Since schools regrettably do not test entering students for these skills, parents may want to seek an eye doctor who will test their child. They should certainly do so if they have any reason to believe the child is lagging in his visual development.

Visual pursuit, or eye tracking, is the ability to follow a moving object with the eyes. The six small muscles attached to the eyeball control the action. Effective visual pursuit requires adequate muscles, and learning how to direct them. When the skill is fully developed, usually not till about age 7, the eyes move smoothly in pursuit of the object. At age 5 their motion is still visibly jerky. Visual tracking is essential to being able to follow what is going on in the classroom and, thus, to paying attention. In order to keep one's place while reading, and to catch a ball, people need good visual eye tracking.

Fixation, the ability to bring both eyes to bear on the same object, must be well advanced. A child whose fixation is poor will have trouble concentrating and keeping attention on what is going on in class. Focusing, or accommodation, which is accomplished by a change in the shape of the lens, should also be well advanced. A child whose focusing is working poorly will be confused by detail when reading. For example, the difference between the words "these" and "those" or "hit" and "kit" might pose a problem. Deficiency in focusing skills often results in poor concentration, headaches and tired eyes.

The small, rapid eye shifts known as saccadic (pronounced suh-CADD-ic) movements will become critically important later on when the child has to read for any length of time. At age 5, before the child is reading, a saccadic deficiency may appear as a difficulty in shifting the eyes from one target to another.

The child's binocular vision must be well developed by the time school starts. This is how children learn to see in three dimension and this is how they locate themselves, and others, in space. A child with poor binocular vision may seem clumsy, and may have trouble putting one block on top of another. They may have trouble pouring water into a cup because of the inability to judge space accurately.

Visual skills typically work together, so a lag in one affects the results obtained by the others. Thus, a child will use clarity of sight, along with eye tracking and binocular vision, to understand what is happening at the front of the room. Often this results in a shift of attention, away from all that is going on around the room, and toward that, which is immediately in front of the student. This student will use saccadic movement and focusing to carry out the teacher's instructions.

These are skills of vision proper. There is yet another skill students need that may seem unrelated to vision. In order to pay attention to what is going on, the student must be able to sit in a comfortable, balanced position. Their sense of posture derives, in part, from messages the eyes send to the body's balancing mechanism. The child has been gradually developing a sense of posture after first learning to crawl, then walk, and finally, run. A child whose posture is not ready for school may be fidgety and often has trouble paying attention.

What we have described here is where a child should be in his or her visual development by the time school starts. Of course, many children are in fact not ready. One estimate based on a very large survey dating from the early 1950s is that two children in every 10 enter school with vision that has not yet reached the stage they need for what they have to do. Our own experience has been that the rate nowadays is much higher, that about four children in 10 are not visually ready when they start school. Recently kindergarten teachers have been reporting that a rising proportion of their entering classes are not ready for school. The number of teachers who make this observation also seems to be rising year by year.

"Why is there such an increased frequency of visual-motor problems in children today compared to 25 years ago?" We have heard that question time and again from veteran kindergarten teachers. We find two major changes in our culture that go a long way toward explaining why so many more children are not visually ready for school.

GAMES

Children's games are constantly changing. Traditional games such as jacks, stoop ball, pickup sticks, marbles, hopscotch, and jump rope are seldom played today. Each of these games, as well as most traditional games of the last century were games that gave children hours and hours of practicing visual-motor coordination. Playing those games functioned as a very important part of children's visual development.

Today electronic and battery-operated toys have largely replaced visual motor coordination games. Manufacturers of these newer electronic games compete for sales by reducing the demand for visual and motor effort by the user. This reduces a lot of practice time that previously was spent developing visual motor skills.

TV, COMPUTERS AND BACK-LIT SCREENS

Today television and computers occupy a large chunk of most children's waking hours. We have no intention of adding to the volumes that have been written on the influence of television on children, so we will confine ourselves to its effects on their visual development. While the field of computer assisted learning is burgeoning in education (and think of all the great iPad learning apps), we believe that the effect of watching excessive TV and sitting in front of computer screens for excessive hours, to be harmful. Television is harmful because it is such a passive activity. In fact, TV is one of the most passive of human activities since it asks nothing of the viewer's visual system beyond a passive stare. And, requires little if anything of the mind. While engaged in passive screen viewing no visual skill growth is accomplished. These critical skills are missed in development as well as development of skills for visual imagination.

At least listening to an iPod requires students to imagine in pictures the scenes that are being described in words or sounds. Creation of visual images must be learned like all other aspects of vision.

If it is true that children watch an average of four hours of television a day, that is a huge loss of time which they might otherwise spend practicing and developing their visual skills. Add to that the practice lost owing to modern children's games, and the learning time taken out of their lives becomes frighteningly large.

Children learn skills the same way everyone does, by practice, and nowadays they are losing a great deal of practice time. Is it any wonder that kindergarten teachers complain that so many children are unprepared, or that so many children in the early grades need some form of remedial therapy to make up for the visual experiences they have never had?

With these examples, a major decision must now be made with regard to these children's educational experiences. Should this child enter first grade or should they remain in kindergarten for another year until visually ready to meet the demands of increasing amounts of close work at school? Is this child ready for the first grade? This should be the real question, and is not asked for the purpose of punishing a child for not being ready for the next grade. Rather, the question needs to be asked in order to properly evaluate whether or not the child is ready to experience success at the first grade level or do they need more time to develop emotional, physical, perceptual and visual skills in order to achieve their potential.

A *New York Times* article (August 20, 2010) written by Pamela Paul entitled "The Littlest Redshirts Sit Out Kindergarten" calls this issue to center stage. In this article the reader is challenged to consider that biological age may be a less reliable indicator for classroom readiness than the "redshirting" of kindergartners.

Redshirting is a term used in athletics at the college level and refers to delayed participation that serves to foster a higher level of participation. The term is not a new one, nor is the concept. Using this reasoning as readiness for participation, an athlete, typically in college, has eligibility spread over a five year span during the four year college curricula. There are many reasons an athlete may become a redshirt. Students may redshirt time to gain practice readiness or so they can mature physically since some sports favor bigger players. Redshirting is beneficial to the team as well as the player.

Using the concept of redshirting for first grade readiness benefits students who are still trying to learn certain/emotional physical skills. This gives them the time they need to advance developmentally before expecting them to achieve in the classroom where other students may be developmentally ahead of them. Since vision is critical to the young student's learning, redshirting is both smart and efficient in determining a fairer pace for the distribution of grade advancement and placement.

REFERENCES

Kavner RS 1985. Kavner Your Child's Vision. New York : Fireside Book.

Wecker NS 2000, Kramer JH, Wisniewski A, Delis DC, Kaplan E. Neuropsychology. Jul;14(3):409-14.

White R 2001. *A precarious balance: Genetic versus environmental risk in the mediation of myopia. British Journal of Ophthalmology. 85:855-60.*

RECOMMENDED READING

Elkind D. *Children and Adolescents. Oxford University Press, USA, 1981.*

Elkind D. *Miseducation: Preschoolers at Risk. New York: Knopf, 1987.*

Elkind D. *The Hurried Child: Growing Up Too Fast Too Soon. Cambridge, MA: Perseus Books, 2001.*

Elkind D. *Power of Play: How Spontaneous, Imaginative Activities Lead to Happier, Healthier Children. Cambridge, MA: Perseus Books, 2007.*

Felton V, Peterson R. *Piaget: A Handbook for Parents and Teachers of Children in the Age of Discovery--Preschool Through Third Grade. Moraga, CA: Victoria Felton, 1976.*

Gesell A, Ilg FL, Bullis GE. *Vision its Development in Infant and Child. Santa Ana, CA: Optometric Extension Program Foundation, 1998.*

Ginsburg H, Opper S. *Piaget's theory of intellectual development. Upper Saddle River, NJ: Prentice-Hall, 1979.*

Mooney CG. *Theories of Childhood:An Introduction to Dewey, Montessori, Erikson, Piaget & Vygotsky. Upper Saddle River, NJ: Pearson/Merrill Prentice Hall, 2005.*

Piaget J. *Origins of Intelligence. New York: W.W. Norton Co., Inc., 1952.*

Ginsburg H, Opper S. *Piaget's Theory of Intellectual Development.*

CHAPTER 4
READING AND VISION IN SCHOOL: WHY SO MANY CHILDREN CAN'T SEE TO READ

Brendan M came to us in April of the year he was in second grade. He was 8 years and 8 months old, and was an unusually bright child. He was in serious trouble however, since he couldn't seem to learn to read. No one could figure out why. Brendan had gotten off to a good start in life, as the healthy child of parents who were both college graduates. He was a happy boy who loved his first school experience in a cooperative playgroup. It was in first grade that the first signs of trouble appeared for him. Despite his natural ability, he wasn't keeping up with his peers when it came to learning to read.

A perceptive nun who was his teacher commented: "I have a sense that Brendan doesn't see what I see. Are you sure he's seeing it right?" A standard eye examination showed him to be mildly farsighted, and thereafter he wore glasses for close work. The glasses, however, did not prove to be of much help in learning to read.

By late in second grade Brendan had fallen far behind. His teacher reported that he was making no progress in reading and writing. He frequently reversed letters. He had "great difficulty with words on a page." In arithmetic, he could not tell when a number was written incorrectly, and he was beginning to reverse two-digit numbers. The teacher could see that he was under stress. He would turn his paper sideways, push away his glasses, and rub his eyes. He was becoming quarrelsome, and would lash out angrily when another child supplied the right answer. Brendan saw a reading tutor, but she reported that he was making no improvement at all. He complained of headaches and discomfort when trying to read or write.

The school psychologist was consulted. His tests showed Brendan to be of considerably above average intelligence, with an IQ of 131. His word use and verbal skills were far advanced for his age level, but his ability to concentrate and pay attention, though average, was below his intellectual capacity. He was eager to do what was expected of him but uncertain that he could meet the demands of school. The psychologist concluded that he Brendan had an" incipient learning disability."

At home, Brendan's parents saw his problems take their toll on his personality. They watched helplessly as their son's once cheerful disposition turned sour. He got into frequent fights, and was frustrated and unhappy. "What's the matter with me?" he would say. Once he told his mother that when he tried to read "the words seem to melt on the page." Now his mother recalled that as a child she had had the same experience: "The words seemed to melt on the page." She wondered if Brendan had inherited some sort of visual problem from her.

Brendan's case is typical of a large number of children. On any given day, there are too many like him in our school system. Once again we refer to the study published by Hokoda (1985) where he clinically documented a 21% rate of binocular vision disorders with accompanying symptomatology found in the school age population. This is one in five children who have the potential for serious reading difficulty due to the inability of their eyes to work together enough for them to see to read without experiencing failure, frustration, anger and impatience with concentration and the ability to focus on what they are reading.

Too many children simply cannot manage reading, and the problem appears to be getting worse as more and more young people are expected to achieve with visual demands at close range than ever before historically.

Five children with visual problems will be found in the average classroom of 25. In the first two grades these children cannot learn to read, and in the later grades they cannot read to learn. They have been classed under various labels, such as "learning disabled," ADD/ADHD, autistic or the most recent category of "executive function deficit disorder" all of which translate as, "We don't know why" or "Your child is different from others their age."

Indeed, no one knows why such a large number of otherwise normal children cannot manage reading. They are normal in the sense that they are not lacking intelligence. The studies of "learning disabled" children show them to be as intelligent as their reading peers.

THE DIVIDED FORM BOARD

On the next page is a test that helps determine whether a child is visually ready to learn. The child is shown the assembled figures, each consisting of two pieces. The figures are then taken apart, and the child is asked to put them together. This test determines whether the child has successfully made the transition from depending on touch for information to the reliance on vision that is necessary for success in school. The transition to visual dominance is usually achieved by the child's seventh year. A first grade student should be able to complete this task in 90 seconds or less.

What happens to these students becomes evident to those who spend a lot of time with young people unsuccessfully struggling to read. We know they started out

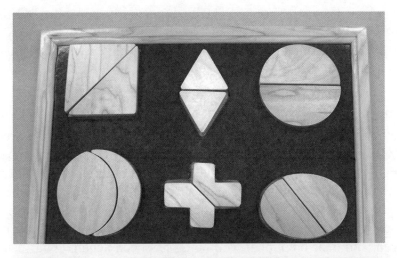

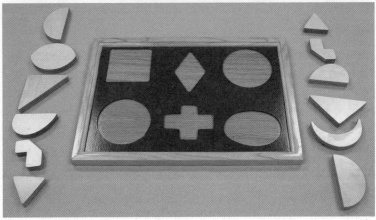

THE DIVIDED FORM BOARD

Shown here is a test that helps determine whether a child is visually ready to learn. The child is shown the assembled figures, each consisting of two pieces, then the figures are taken apart and the child is asked to put them together. This test determines whether the child has successfully made the transition from depending on touch for information to the reliance on vision that is necessary for success in school. The transition to visual dominance is usually achieved by the child's seventh year. A first-grade child should be able to complete this task in 90 seconds or less.

at school happy and very eager to learn at age 5 or 6. They possessed the natural curiosity that is part of what defines us as human beings. Then, when confronted with having to learn to read in school, they start to inexplicably struggle with many aspects of their home and school life. They sense that they are failing repeatedly. They are intellectually ready to learn, but the primary path to learning is through reading. So this first experience of school, of the world of organized education, is not unfolding very well. These bright, eager and enthusiastic students react as one does to failure.

The big question here is whether or not the child is physiologically ready for learning and reading. For example, a child may be able to converse and interact at a 9 year old level, but they may not be physiologically ready for learning and reading at the first grade level. They may not be visually, binocularly, perceptually, motorically, and or vestibularly ready for the school experience. In other words, they are physiologically not ready. We may need to stop and focus on the visual, binocular and or perceptual aspects of the child's development.

Children faced with the obstacle of underdeveloped vision start to give up on learning. By age 9 they seem to hate school because reading is way too frustrating. They often appear to be hyperactive, and may even disrupt the classroom, or, at the other extreme, withdraw silently into a corner. In time, they may learn to read well enough to get by in school and, later, in life, but precious years have been irretrievably lost. The continued failure leads to loss of self confidence, as well as psychological and emotional complications. By this time they have learned to perform below their potential, in many cases, far below. By now, their personality has changed, and their emotional well being has been negatively affected. Sadly, these may be lifelong alterations. The cost to the student and his or her family is high, as it also is to society.

Why can't these children learn? Vision therapy is not a panacea, and unlike the quick conclusions often drawn when labeling kids with attention deficit spectrum terms, vision therapy does not claim to solve all reading problems or cure children with learning disabilities. However, decades of scientific documentation coupled with a high success rate in clinical studies, points us toward vision therapy as a solution to a many of these issues.

Vision disorders are found to exist in a very large number of cases of learning disability. Statistics prove this repeatedly. One such study (Mohney, McKenzie, Capo, Nusz, Mrazek, Diehl 2008) showed that close to 75% of reading-disabled children have a vision disorder. This compares to 22% for children with no reading problem. Other surveys verify these results. Brian Mohney, MD, (Mayo Clinic 2008) of the Mayo Clinic published results of a study in the journal, *Pediatrics*. The results showed that children with divergent strabismus were three times more likely to develop a psychiatric disorder than children with normal eye alignment. It was also proven that patients with intermittent divergent strabismus were more likely to have mental health disorders and thoughts of suicide or homicide.

Simply put, the evidence is overwhelming, and it is time for the importance of vision to learning to be publicly recognized where it matters the most, in school. As one optometrist, Tole Greenstein, put it, "Those who deny that vision plays a major role in learning problems rely on the evidence of the standard eye examination. The standard eye exam only tests eye sight at close and distance measures along with checking for astigmatism, all of which deal with distortions in the shape of the eyeball. That, along with a check for disease or a turned eye, is all that shows up on the standard eye exam."

There is no greater rate of learning disability than that observed in children with refractive error. In the case of myopia, the opposite is true. Nearsighted children tend to be better readers. The conventional image of the bespectacled bookworm finds confirmation in the statistics. Most cases of myopia are the result of the eyeball adapting to the stress of prolonged nearpoint work. Scientific and clinical evidence show this longtime theory to have been true all along. Good readers read more, and in so doing, are more likely to become more nearsighted with each year of intense close work. The eye screening given to many children in school usually falls short of what is necessary for a complete vision evaluation, revealing less than 5% of visual problems.

Visual disorders found in so many learning disabled children are those who have their causes beyond the retina. The problems are in vision and visual perception. As we saw in the previous chapter, children start school before they have fully learned to use their visual systems. They lack the background of experience from which perception is based. They are not fully able to interpret the evidence of their senses, and their thinking processes are not mature. According to Jean Piaget, the great Swiss epistemologist and student of child development, all children must pass through stages of cognitive development in which their ways of thinking are distinctively different from those of adults. The picture of a child thinking like a miniature adult, or smaller version of an adult, is unacceptable!

Only after around age 11, do children begin to reason as adults do, and a great many never make the last transition. Thirty percent of students still need to make the transition when they reach 14, which means they enter high school without the capacity for adult reasoning and problem solving skills that high school requires.

TWO KINDS OF VISION PROBLEMS

Vision problems in school age children fall into two broad categories besides the refractive errors treated by standard eye doctors. One category consists of physiological disorders of vision proper, problems in how the eyes function as directed by the brain.

- **Binocular Fusion** is the ability to bring the two eyes together so that their images fuse and integrate, and to maintain that fusion comfortably for sustained periods of time while reading or working on a computer terminal.

- **Focus Accommodation** is the ability to see clearly at a fixed distance and to shift focus quickly, with instantaneous clarity from one distance to another. An example of focus accommodation is when one looks from desk to blackboard.

- **Fixation** is the ability to locate a target and stabilize the eyes so that the images of the target fall on the retina at the most desirable angle.

- **Eye Movement** is the ability to move the eyes quickly, accurately, and in precise coordination. An example is the ability to follow along while reading or following a moving ball.

The second category consists of problems in visual perception, or how the child uses information from the eyes.

- **Visual Verbal Match** is the ability to match information from hearing words spoken, with visually recognizing and seeing words that are written. This is what is needed as one is learning to read.

- **Figure Ground Perception** is the ability to discern that which matters and disregard surrounding irrelevant information. An example would be concentrating on one problem among many on an arithmetic worksheet.

- **Directionality In Space** is the ability to tell up from down or left from right, for example, seeing the difference between b and d, or "was" and "saw."

- **Visual Form Perception** is the ability to recognize differences in shape, for example, the shapes of letters.

- **Visual Motor Coordination** is the ability to coordinate vision and body actions, for example, eyes and hand in writing or catching a ball.

- **Visual Imagery** is the ability to picture something that is not physically visible at the moment, for example, in scanning a word in the mind's eye to see if it looks properly spelled.

Before reaching adulthood, children perceive the world differently. They are not miniature adults. They interpret evidence according to different mental standards that proceed in predictable patterns. Up to about seven, for example, children tend to believe anything they see. They are an excellent audience for a magician: they believe the rabbit really came out of the hat because that is what they saw and they have not yet learned to interpret the evidence of their eyes.

Small children are dominated by their visual perception and make great candidates for being easily tricked. Take for example a bag of m&m's® candy. When given a choice between a large 8 oz. size Hershey bar versus a 8 oz. bag of m&m's® small children usually pick the m&m's because they think that they are picking the 'bigger' choice because there are more pieces!

Another example involves the principle of conservation. Pour a given amount of water from a tall, narrow beaker into one that is short and broad in the presence of a 5 year old child. The 5 year old will invariably pick one beaker or the other as containing or having contained more water. Or, press a piece of putty into two pieces of exactly the same size in which one is different in shape. Again, the child will pick one shape as larger than others. Only later, again around age 7, will thinking develop to the point where children can perceive that different shapes can contain (or "conserve") the same quantity. Many children have not yet established vision as their dominant sense, the sense on which they primarily rely for information. They still need to touch an object to grasp its reality—an obvious handicap in the classroom, where they must understand actions that take place beyond their arms' length.

Most children, as we well know, learn to read nonetheless, but a substantial minority is just not ready for what is a difficult undertaking in the best of circumstances. Dr. Arnold Gesell, director of the child development clinic at Yale University, pioneered the work on vision of children, estimating that from a quarter to a half of them were not "visually ready" when they enter first grade. Children who are not visually ready will be less observant, remember less, learn less, be confused and frustrated and generally be less efficient at what they do. Again, many of them will overcome the handicap and learn to read. But for many others the gap is too great. They will join the ranks of the learning disabled. Their visual problems remain unnoticed, and indeed, they often do better than average on the Snellen chart. As Dr. William M. Ludlam, director of a learning disability clinic at Pacific University observed, "They'd make great buffalo hunters, but not good students."

The problems developmental optometrists find in such children fall into two broad categories, with a bundle of related problems within each category. One group consists of physiological disorders of vision proper. The child cannot move his eyes well, or cannot focus quickly and accurately. They also cannot use their eyes as a team for binocular vision.

The other category includes disorders of perception which manifest in the way children can or cannot use their vision. An obvious example is poor eye-hand coordination that makes it hard to form letters with a pencil. Spelling becomes difficult as does putting thoughts on paper. Another problem that emerges is the inability to connect in the mind with what is seen and heard. Children struggling with these types of problems have difficulty translating the teacher's verbal instruction into written work on paper.

Still another problem in this category of vision disorders has to do with what is called "directionality" or the ability to tell left from right. Children with directionality problems cannot tell b from d, or p from g (letter pairs involving left-right orientation), nor can they understand what is intended when told to move their eyes and hands from left to right across the page

Although children typically show problems in both areas, the emphasis shifts with changing requirements of school. In the first two grades, disorders of perception are usually more important to the child as a handicap to learning. The case of Marygrace K is an example of a child with this type of problem.

Marygrace *was a pretty little girl at 5 years and 9 months old. Three weeks into first grade at a Catholic academy where she had attended kindergarten, it appeared that she might be sent back to repeat kindergarten. She scored in an average range on intelligence tests. She showed an IQ of 100. She did poorly in kindergarten and was already not doing well in first grade.*

Her teacher described Marygrace as a hyperactive child with a short attention span. Her mother said she was clumsy. When she came to us this child

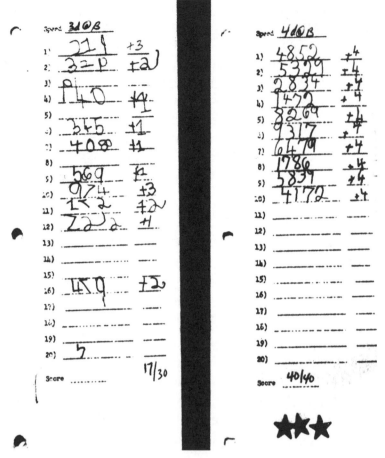

MARYGRACE'S WORK

Above are Marygrace's scores in a test of her ability to absorb and reproduce visual information. An instrument called the tachistoscope flashes on a screen, groups of numbers, which the patient tries to reproduce from memory. The first column shows Marygrace's score when the instrument displayed groups of three digits, showing each group for one-tenth of a second. In this test, before her therapy, she got 17 of 30 correct. The second column shows the result when the tachistoscope showed her groups of four digits for one-hundredth of a second. In this more difficult test, after therapy, Marygrace got 40 of 40 correct. Note also the great improvement in her handwriting in only eight months.

already seemed to be marked by failure. She looked down instead of looking people in the eye and she did not smile much.

Our examination showed Marygrace to be far behind in the development of her perceptual skills. Her ability to copy what she saw was about eighteen months behind her age, a potentially disastrous lag at that time of life. She also had trouble recognizing and recording digits flashed on a screen by an instrument called a tachistoscope.

MARYGRACE'S WORK

Above are Marygrace's scores in a test of her ability to absorb and reproduce visual information. An instrument called the tachistoscope flashes groups of

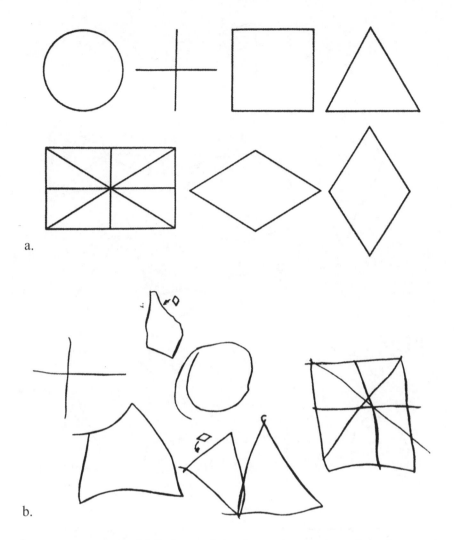

a.

b.

numbers on a screen which the patient then tries to reproduce from memory. The first column shows Marygrace's score when the instrument displayed groups of three digits, showing each group for one-tenth of a second. Before therapy, Marygrace got 17 of 30 correct on this test. The second column shows the result when the tachistoscope showed her groups of four digits for one-hundredth of a second each. This is a difficult test, and Marygrace scored 40 out of 40 correct after undergoing vision therapy. Additional improvement was observed in her handwriting. These therapeutic advances occurred over an eight month time frame.

Above are Marygrace's drawings in what is called the Winter Haven Visual Copy Forms Test. The patient is shown the whole group of geometrical figures (a), then is shown the individual figures one by one and asked to copy them. This process tests the patient's eye-hand coordination and his or her ability to organize and use spatial information. In the first two tests, before (b) and during (c) therapy, Marygrace's performance is below average for her age.

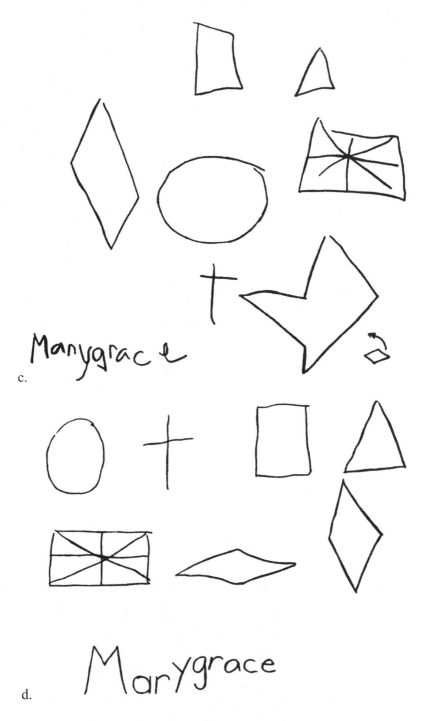

c. Manygrace

d. Marygrace

In the last test (d) her skills have advanced in age level by 24 months in only 9 months' time.

Marygrace had virtually no understanding of left and right; she could not follow an instruction to move an arm or leg on one or the other side. She could not bounce a ball with one hand, then the other, which is unusual at that age. Tests for other perceptual skills all showed her performing considerably below her age and intelligence levels.

Marygrace started on a program of treatment that was to last 10 months. The therapy provided her with concentrated practice in all the skills in which she was deficient. Believing it essential to offer her success rather than still more failure, we began by reinforcing and perfecting those skills, which she could, to some degree, handle. Then, as soon as possible, but always building on success, we moved her on to gradually more advanced skills.

Marygrace's treatment was successful. Far from being put back, she performed exceedingly well in first grade. She was one of the best students. She went on to do equally well in second grade. When she was tested at the beginning of second grade 10 months after we first examined her the difference was dramatic. Over the full range of perceptual skills, Marygrace tested above, and in some categories, far above, the average for her age. In no case did she test below average. She no longer had trouble with left and right and she could now bounce a ball. Her scholastic achievement scores were on a third grade level. In less than 12 months she had advanced by at least two years.

Marygrace was doing well in school and, moreover, she seemed like a different child. Now she smiled and looked us in the eye. Her manner was self assured. She even seemed more concerned about her personal appearance. Would Marygrace have caught up to her class anyway, without our therapy? Unfortunately, the experience of many other children shows that the mere passage of time does not guarantee that the child will gain the skills she is lacking: the right kind of experience is also necessary. In any event the question in practice does not arise. In a perfect world, children like Marygrace would not be asked to read until they were visually ready.

As we all know, the world is not perfect. School is a large-scale institution in which children must keep up with the group. The group will not wait for the Marygrace's of our world. When she falls behind she will be branded a failure, in her own eyes as well as those of others.

DOES YOUR CHILD NEED HELP WITH VISUAL SKILLS?

A Checklist for Parents

What follows are two lists of questions for parents of school age children.

The first list of questions is about urgent signs of possible visual problems. If the answer to any one of these 11 questions is yes, the child should get a full evaluation of visual skills.

1. Does your child see double?
2. Does she get frequent headaches?

3. Does he have a short attention span while reading?

4. Does she frequently lose her place while reading, or use a finger as a pointer?

5. Is he in the lowest reading group?

6. Does she have very poor handwriting?

7. Does he avoid reading?

8. Does she say that the print in a book is blurred, or that it blurs in and out of focus?

9. Does he have difficulty seeing the chalkboard in school?

10. Does she make frequent reversals, such as "was" for "saw" or 34 for 43?

11. Does one of your child's eyes turn in or out?

This second list of questions is about less severe signs of troubled vision. If the answer to five or more of these questions is yes, the child's visual skills should be evaluated.

1. Does your child hold the book very close to the eyes (7 or 8 inches) while reading or writing?

2. Does she have her head turned while working at a desk?

3. Does he rest his head on his arm while reading or writing?

4. Does she cover one eye while reading?

5. Does he squint while doing close visual work?

6. Does she consistently show poor posture while doing close work?

7. Does he move his head back and forth while reading instead of just his eyes?

8. Does her reading homework take her longer than it should?

9. Does he report that print becomes blurry after prolonged reading, though at first it was clear?

10. Does she complain of words or letters running together?

11. Does he rub his eyes or blink excessively during or after close work?

12. Do her eyes appear red during or after reading?

13. Does he lose his place when moving his gaze from desk to chalkboard or when copying from text to notebook?

14. Does her writing slant up or down on the page, or is the spacing irregular between words or letters?

15. Does your child repeatedly omit or add or substitute small words while reading or writing?

16. Does he reread or skip words or lines without knowing he is doing it?

17. Does she fail to recognize the same word in the next sentence?

18. Does his reading comprehension decrease the longer he reads?

19. Does she have trouble sustaining concentration on any deskwork?

20. Does he misalign digits in columns of numbers?

21. Is she slow at copying?

22. Does he seem unable to stay on ruled lines when writing?

23. Does she turn or rotate the paper in order to draw lines in different directions?

24. Does he consistently have trouble putting thoughts on paper (for example, writing a letter describing a vacation trip)?

25. Does he have difficulty catching or hitting a ball?

26. Does she have difficulty closing buttons or tying shoelaces?

27. Does he have difficulty distinguishing left from right?

28. Does she get carsick?

A couple of years of repeated failure will do considerable damage to such a child. Even if she does catch up in her perceptual skills, she may never catch up academically, because her appetite for learning has been stunted and in the effort to get by in school she has formed poor scholastic habits that will outlast their cause. The same is true of children whose superior natural ability enables them to keep up despite a lag in their perceptual development. They will keep up but they will not work up to their potential: a child of 130 IQ, let us say, will do average work when he could do far better.

We believe that in both cases the cost in lost potential and human unhappiness of waiting for nature to do it, which will probably never happen, is far too great when another way is available. Unfortunately, children with perceptual problems seldom are brought to us as early as they should be. The issue is not as clear as it is when the child has an obviously visual problem. Usually other professionals are already involved, for, when a child with apparently good eyesight can't seem to learn, one is not likely to turn first to an optometrist. It is true that sometimes we succeed in removing the perceptual problem and the child still does not learn. Children who master the perceptual skills but still do not learn are suffering from some other impediment that must be resolved, if indeed it can be, by someone in another field though it may still have been necessary first to remove the perceptual problem.

*When we examined **Brendan**, we found that he was suffering from several related disorders of vision. His complaints of headaches when he tried to read or write were understandable. Brendan literally couldn't read. Any sustained close work was painful for his eyes, and he was mildly farsighted, although corrected with glasses. With or without glasses, however, he could not make his eyes work as a team. He could not make the two pictures his eyes saw fuse into a single stable image, and his binocular vision was poor. He could not hold his eyes in focus; that was why, as he told his mother, "the words seem to melt on the page." He also showed symptoms of perceptual immaturity, but these were mild compared to his visual disorders.*

We started Brendan on a course of vision therapy that lasted for 30 sessions in our office, plus a set of supplementary home exercises. The purpose of the therapy is to create situations in which the brain is induced to give the right messages to the eyes. To repeat an earlier comparison, this is much like learning a skill such as touch typing.

Like touch typing, it takes a lot of practice before it becomes second nature. The visual situations are created with the use of lenses and prisms and various kinds of instruments, some simple, some elaborate. Some of the routines are games that will challenge a patient, whether child or adult.

By about halfway through the course we could observe the improvement in Brendan's visual skills. By the time he began third grade he was finished with his therapy. His visual skills were normal.

The scholastic results of Brendan's therapy can be easily summarized. He started with us late in second grade. By the middle of third grade he was

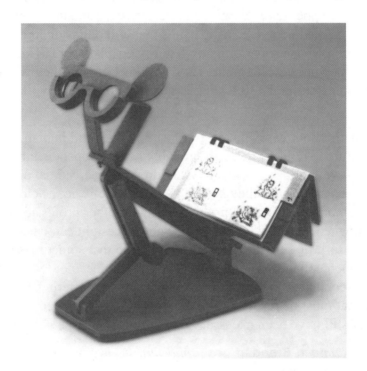

TESTING BINOCULAR SKILLS I

The cheiroscope, shown in the photo, is used both to test and to improve the ability to integrate information from the two eyes. The instrument presents separate images to each eye. The patient is asked to trace with each hand the image that is seen. The tracings reproduced here show the progress in therapy of an adult patient suffering from intermittent divergent strabismus; her left eye turned out. In the center in each case is the image she was asked to reproduce; on each side are what she respectively traced with her left and right hands. In the first tracing, the patient saw nothing at all on the left side and on the right she was able to reproduce only part of the object. In the second she was able to reproduce on the left side, and by the end of therapy, five months later, her binocular skills had improved to the point where she was able accurately to reproduce a clown holding a pig, an image far more complex than those she had previously been tested on.

Photo courtesy of Bernell Corporation, South Bend, Indiana

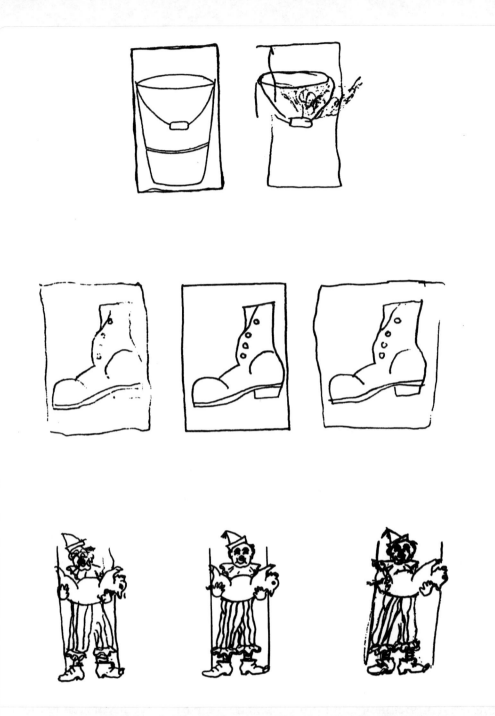

reading at grade level. That same year Brendan won the class reading prize. His attitude was transformed. His parents reported that he was once again the cheerful, self-confident boy he had been before his visual troubles got in his way. Brendan has since graduated from an Ivy League university. It is worth noting that Brendan had received no other form of intervention during the time he was having his vision therapy. He did not have any treatment from a psychologist or reading specialist.

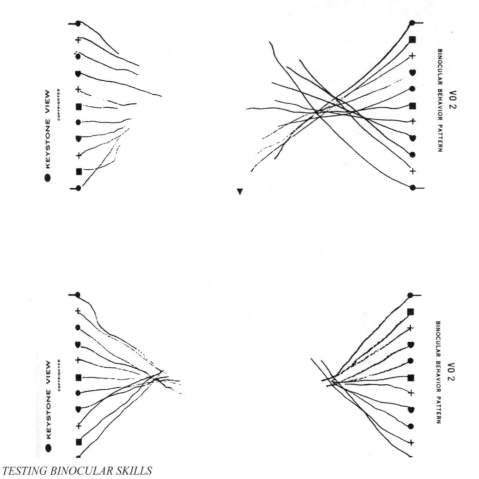

TESTING BINOCULAR SKILLS

The tracings reproduced here were made with the cheiroscope, the instrument shown on page 58, which displays separate images to each eye. The patient is asked to draw lines simultaneously with her left and right hands so that they appear to meet. The first line starts at the top left for the left hand and at the bottom right for the right hand, the next line one down at left and one up at right, and so on. The patient, who suffered from intermittent strabismus (her left eye turned in), was unable in the first drawing to complete the lines on the left side. She tried to compensate by extending the right lines. Six months later she was able to bring the lines together, demonstrating a great improvement in her binocular vision.

In the later years of grade school the demands on children's vision increase dramatically, and the primary problems we encounter are disorders of the visual skills. In the first two grades the child is learning the code that is reading, and his problems, if any, are usually in his visual perception. He is not called on to do much reading for information. Beginning in third grade, and increasing steadily thereafter, he is expected to read to learn: the skill must be second nature; for the first time in his life he must be able to read for sustained periods. The type in his books is much smaller than the letters on the blocks in first grade, and he has to keep his mind on it for much longer.

In its demand on vision, reading a chapter is radically different from reading a line. The child now confronts the intense close work that A. M. Skeffington, the father of modern vision therapy, called "an affront and insult to the natural and primitive use of eyesight."

Now even minor flaws in vision (flaws our hunter ancestors, with their eyes focused on the horizon, would never even notice) can prove an insurmountable handicap. These flaws, which typically involve the ability to make the eyes work together, begin to show up when the child has to read the fine print. A good example is "saccadic movements." When we read, our eyes do not glide smoothly across the page; they move in a series of very short, rapid, very precise jumps, several times a second and several times a line. Several times a second, the eyes must focus, read, jump, refocus, and read. Flaws in these skills manifest themselves, not in the inability to read, but in the growing discomfort of reading over time. The child can read a line but not a chapter, because his or her eyes are not tracking words properly. When this child is called on to read aloud, they feel embarrassed, often repeating, omitting or stumbling over even familiar words. This child is likely to have trouble copying from the board and in sustaining attention. The symptoms the child reports often show the wearing effects of attempting to read with imperfect vision. About 40% of the school-age patients we see report that by late in the school day they are seeing double and many say, like Brendan, that the print seems to swim in and out of focus.

Robbie C *did fairly well in the first three grades. He was considered a bit slow; reading below grade level, but not far below. His teachers said he was a "very nice boy." The roof fell in when Robbie reached fifth grade. His teacher summoned his mother and told her Robbie was "learning disabled" and was a disciplinary problem. She wanted the once nice boy out of her class-room. He was now two years behind in reading and arithmetic The school threatened to hold him back so Robbie's parents took him to a psychologist, who found during testing, that Robbie was dropping whole phrases when he read aloud. This discovery eventually brought Robbie in for vision therapy. We found that he suffered from intermittent strabismus: one eye drifted out, came back, drifted out again. This condition is particularly hard for the visual system, because the brain cannot make a lasting adjustment as it can if the eye is consistently turned. He was one or two years behind in his perceptual skills. He said he suffered from eyestrain and that his sight often blurred.*

After Robbie had been in vision therapy for nine months, clinical tests showed that his vision was normal. His drifting eye was straight. His skills were now at his age level. In school his arithmetic began to improve right away while reading improved more slowly. In the next three years Robbie picked up the equivalent of five years in his schoolwork and caught up. Robbie's life changed in other ways. Before his therapy he had been a clumsy boy who avoided sports and whose leg turned in when he ran. By the end of the third year after his therapy he had become much more physical and was an above-average soccer player.

Visual disorders tend to run in families. No one knows if this means the disorders have genetic causes or whether they result from family environment or, perhaps, some of each. Still, the fact remains that if one member of the family has troubled vision, there is a good chance others will also.   We were not surprised when Robbie's parents brought his younger brother to us.

> **Keith C**'s *parents noticed from his birth that one eye was somewhat turned in.   It was only slightly turned and, since it did not seem to bother him, they did nothing about it. Keith did very well in school. He was well ahead of grade level in all his skills, and he always got good grades. But, his mother thought he was a very aggressive, high-strung boy who couldn't sit still and who "seemed to be churning inside."*

> *She brought Keith to us to check his vision. Like his older brother, Keith suffered from intermittent strabismus, but in his case the eye turned in rather than out. Maintaining binocular vision was a constant struggle for him. We suggested vision therapy and we prescribed dual-focus lenses for his glasses.*

> *After a year of therapy, Keith's turned eye was straight. His visual and perceptual skills test at normal levels. He was much calmer. "The tension has gone out of his life," his mother said and his severe headaches went away when he remembered to wear his glasses, or contact lenses.*

Many parents of children who, like Keith, suffer from strabismus have followed an eye doctor's recommendation to have a surgeon operate on the turned eye. Yet it has long been known that this surgery usually produces only a cosmetic result while the untreated vision problems remain.

Sometimes vision therapy succeeds in solving the immediate problem but has to be reinforced later on. This is more likely to be observed when the visual system is still developing and when the demands on vision are changing radically as they do in the later grades of elementary school. Such was the case with Lindsay G, whom we met in the last chapter when she was four and wearing a patch to treat her lazy left eye.

> **Lindsey** *did well in school from the beginning. Her grades were well above average and she was well above grade level in reading and arithmetic. She was a promising young athlete. All went well for the first three grades. But in fourth grade Lindsay began to have serious problems. Her schoolwork continued to be good, but the increase in reading she had to do was a strain for her. Her mother had to help with homework by reading alternate pages aloud. Lindsay had no trouble reading as such, it was just the amount of it that was hard for her. She pushed aside her glasses, saying they were of no use to her, and rubbed her eyes. She complained of headaches as she had years earlier. She put her face down very close to her work, and when watching television would sit within a foot or two of the set. Her eye practitioner said her lazy left eye was once more not working for her, and he*

recommended vision therapy. We found that the great difference between the sight in one eye and in the other was causing trouble now that a lot of reading was demanded of her.

Three months of therapy made a change in Lindsay that was quick and dramatic. We succeeded in equalizing the sight in her two eyes. As a result, her headaches were greatly diminished and she was no longer rubbing her eyes. Her grades, always good, now shot up into the upper 90s, and she was on the honor roll although, her mother said, she needed less time for study. She was enjoying reading again and was taking books out of the library. She no longer asked her mother for help in getting through her reading.

Lindsay's mother felt her daughter was once again the happy child she had been before fourth grade. Lindsey even started playing vision therapist on weekends, asking her friends to pose as her patients. She was looking forward to the next summer's tennis season.

Once again we must remind the reader that vision therapy should never be viewed as a magic bullet or simple panacea for problems in children that are complex and may also involve trouble with reading. Vision therapists are the first to raise awareness for the complex nature of behavioral, perceptual, personality and learning problems that are complex. The inability to read has many roots, and vision therapy as a profession and vision therapists as clinicians do not have all the answers.

Not all reading problems can be attributed to visual disorders, nor does vision therapy always succeed. Here we should note that success in our field is not an either/or proposition like treating a contagion: either you still have the bug or you don't. Like practicing a skill, vision therapy need not have all-or-nothing results: you can improve your vision a little, quite a bit, or a great deal. So we find that while a few children will drop out or make little noticeable improvement, the great majority end up with visual skills that are at or above normal.

Good vision does not guarantee good reading. Some children whose vision therapy is successful may still need other forms of help from a psychologist or a reading specialist in order to catch up in reading. This is especially true, if the child has had a relatively long record of failure before his/her therapy. When a child is profoundly discouraged about school and learning, the road back is not easy, and clearing away a visual obstacle is not all that must be done to rescue the child.

Readers should be aware that vision therapy may not correct a reading problem; reading specialists are the experts at teaching others to read well. There is a substantial amount of research that confirms that vision therapy improves reading comprehension by enabling students learning to read the ability to concentrate so they can better assimilate and process what they read.

A study completed and published by Dr. Seiderman (Seiderman 1980), evaluating 36 children identified as learning disabled with visual and perceptual disorders revealed that the experimental group of children who received individual programming in visual and perceptual development made significant gains in reading as compared to the control group. Both groups received individualized reading assistance. Results showed that the Informal Reading Inventory (Temple University), and the Word Reading and Paragraph Meaning subtests of the Stanford Achievement Tests, along with the actual classroom reading levels were all statistically significant.

Results of another study of sixth grade students with below average reading scores found that providing vision therapy significantly improved both attention and thus, reading comprehension.

The study, "Research Confirms Vision Therapy Can Improve Reading Comprehension" was published in 2003 in the *Journal of Learning Disabilities*. Researcher, Dr. Harold Solan documented the role that vision therapy plays in successfully improving a child's ability to read. As a result, the child's overall attention in the classroom noticeably improves. According to Dr. Solan, the findings of this landmark supports previous research that found visual attention and eye movement abilities greatly contribute to reading ability, comprehension and attention. Again and again, scientific evidence repeatedly confirms that visual attention may be improved through vision therapy whereby improving reading comprehension. Once again, Dr. Solan's work objectively reaffirms the benefits of optometric vision therapy performed by qualified developmental optometrists.

Another analogy that fits Brendan's case is as follows: imagine that you must get through a great deal of printed material for tomorrow's meeting and you have a splitting headache. You take some aspirin. The headache goes away. You still haven't read all that fine print, but now you feel able to tackle it. Like the aspirin, vision therapy can serve as the first step, making the rest possible. This is not only a big step forward, but one of critical importance. Being able to sustain visual concentration will improve one's comprehension.

REFERENCES

Hokoda SC 1985. *General binocular dysfunctions in an urban optometry clinic. J Am Optom Assoc 56:560-3.*

Mayo Clinic 2008. *Eye Divergence in Children Triples Risk of Mental Illness. November 26. http://www.mayoclinic.org/news2008-rst/5103.html.*

Mohney BG, McKenzie JA, Capo JA, Nusz KJ, Mrazek D, Diehl NN, 2008. *Mental illness in young adults who had strabismus as children. Pediatrics 122:1033–8.*

Seiderman A 1980. *Optometric vision therapy- results of a demonstration project with a learning disabled population. Journal of American Optometric Association 51:489-492,*

Solan H. 2003. *Research Confirms Vision Therapy Can Improve Reading Comprehension. http://www.visionhelp.com/vh_resources_06.html. Last accessed: July 11, 2012.*

RECOMMENDED READING

Furth HG. *Piaget for Teachers. Englewood Cliffs, NJ: Prentice Hall, 1970.*

Doidge N. *The Brain that Changes Itself. New York: Viking Penguin, 2007.*

Sacks O. *The Mind's Eye. New York: Alfred A. Knopf, 2010*

CHAPTER 5
ADD, ADHD OR CI?

"The eye sees only what the mind is prepared to comprehend." Henri Bergson

Why can't my child concentrate? The teacher thinks it might be attention deficit disorder (ADD) or attention deficit hyperactivity disorder (ADHD) and it seems like the pediatrician is listening to the teacher. I am confused and I cannot understand what has happened to my otherwise happy child. A child struggling with convergence insufficiency disorder (CI) may complain of the following while using computers, playing handheld video toys, reading or doing any other type of close work:

- Can't concentrate
- Mind wanders
- Short attention span
- Can't sustain focus
- Headaches
- Skipping words or lines when reading
- Trouble remembering what was read
- Avoidance of concentrated work or study that is within 18 inches of the face
- Eyestrain (especially during or after reading)
- Double vision.
- Blurred vision or print in book or on computer screen goes in and out of focus
- Lack of patience with detailed tasks

What happens when health problems share common sets of symptoms? What happens when patients, parents or doctors see an overlapping pattern of symptoms shared by different diseases? What happens when symptoms from one disorder are confused with identical symptoms of a different disorder? These are the questions that this chapter addresses and the aim is to empower families to ask the right questions about ADD and ADHD in order to be sure that nothing is missed and nothing is misdiagnosed and that things unfold in ways that are best for their child. On the next page is a compare and contrast chart with the shared symptoms of vision problems and attention deficit disorders. Notice the overlap. Symptoms of both CI and ADD/ADHD are bold faced.

VISION PROBLEMS

- Has difficulty with attention to details
- *makes careless mistakes*
- *is easily distracted by stimuli around them*
- forgets to do daily tasks
- *has difficulty concentrating*
- loses things
- *has difficulty sustaining attention*
- often does not listen when spoken to directly
- *mind seems to wander*
- does not follow through on tasks and often does not finish tasks
- has difficulty organizing self and work
- *avoids activity that requires sustained mental effort*
- *avoids activity that requires concentration*
- looses things and is forgetful
- fidgets or squirms instead of paying attention
- is impatient: does not like to wait for their turn
- is restless
- talks excessively and interrupts others

ATTENTION DEFICITS

- Has difficulty with attention to details
- *makes careless mistakes*
- *is easily distracted by stimuli around them*
- forgets to do daily tasks
- *has difficulty concentrating*
- loses things
- *has difficulty sustaining attention*
- often does not listen when spoken to directly
- *mind seems to wander*
- does not follow through on tasks and often does not finish tasks
- has difficulty organizing self and work
- *avoids activity that requires sustained mental effort*
- *avoids activity that requires concentration*
- looses things and is forgetful
- fidgets or squirms instead of paying attention
- is impatient: does not like to wait for their turn
- is restless
- talks excessively and interrupts others

Consider that there is a significant amount of overlap between childhood vision problems and attention deficit symptoms, wouldn't it simply make good sense to rule out vision disorders by completing a comprehensive visual examination, which must include elaborate testing for binocular dysfunction on ALL children being considered for the diagnosis of ADD or ADHD. This is particularly important because the vision exam has objective criteria for determining a diagnosis while ADD and ADHD syndromes do not. Wouldn't it make good sense to perform a complete comprehensive visual examination in order to conform to modern diagnostic methods? Wouldn't it be wise to complete a comprehensive visual examination on these patients simply as a matter of good clinical practice?

Why is the vision exam, more often than not, ignored? Who is doing the testing? Who is doing the diagnosing? If a vision exam is performed and a vision problem is picked up, why is the patient and family not informed of the benefits of opto-metric vision therapy performed by a developmental optometrist? Without all of the facts of a complete accurate diagnosis, with fully informed parents, consent is not possible. This bears repeating:

Without full accurate information given to parents, consent to treatment is not possible. Information on the benefits of vision therapy, along with referral to a qualified developmental/behavioral doctor of optometry is good clinical protocol for a child found to have a visual developmental or binocular problem. Omitting to reveal this information to parents is to deny parents the ability to make informed choices and give autonomous authorization on their child's behalf. Once again, checking for *20/20 IS NOT ENOUGH* and a prescription for glasses to correct to 20/20 eyesight does not solve the problem. The behavioral or functional visual problem is in the brain and this is where vision therapy can help.

For a teacher to send a note home, or have a parent teacher meeting and tell parents "I think your child has ADD/ADHD and needs medication," is for the teacher to accept the liability of practicing medicine without a license. A license to teach is to do just that, it is not a license to diagnose medical problems, nor does it permit the teacher to "medicalize" a child's behavior by using diagnostic terms. One sometimes must wonder whether the drug is prescribed for the child or the teacher's best interest.

Historically, health care has moved away from subjective criteria for diagnosis toward scientific criteria and evidence based diagnostic tools, which are objective. For example, dentists used to smell a bad tooth to determine if a root canal was needed. Not all dentists had the same ability to smell infection, so some patients were healed while others stayed in pain. Today, the modern method is to culture infections and take X-rays to determine if treatment is needed.

Another example is the definition of death and how it has changed over the decades. A century ago, without sensitive tools to determine life inside a person who was non-responsive, a person was pronounced dead when the doctor said so. A half decade ago, the criteria for death was that there was no heart beat and no breathing. Today, we might start CPR on a person in this category and life supports might augment a medical team to save their life. Today, we have tools that pick up heart-beats and breathing so fine that they are imperceptible to our eyes and ears. Death is determined through objective criteria and not someone's opinion.

So too is the need for objectivity in diagnosing ADD, ADHD, Asperger syndrome and autism. A diagnosis of any of these brain-based spectrum disorders is simply incomplete if it does not include a comprehensive visual exam by a qualified behavioral optometrist.

According to the guidelines established by the American Psychiatric Association *Diagnostic and Statistical Manual of Mental Disorders (DSM-IV-TR)* criteria, six or more of the following signs of inattention need to be present, for at least six months, to a point that is disruptive and inappropriate for the child's developmental level, in order to be considered to have an attention deficit spectrum disorder. Since there are no objective measurable diagnostic tests for ADD/ADHD, the general rule is that if people interviewed about the child can identify a minimum of six items from the list, then they are considered to have an attention spectrum disorder. The list is as follows and again we have highlighted the overlapping objective symptoms of developmental vision problems in children, hidden amongst the subjective symptoms of ADD and ADHD

- *has difficulty with attention to details*
- *makes careless mistakes*
- *is easily distracted by stimuli around them*
- forgets to do daily tasks
- *has difficulty concentrating*
- loses things
- *has difficulty sustaining attention*
- often does not listen when spoken to directly
- *mind seems to wander*
- does not follow through on tasks and often does not finish tasks
- has difficulty organizing self and work
- *avoids activity that requires sustained mental effort*
- *avoids activity that requires concentration*
- *fidgets or squirms instead of paying attention*
- is impatient, does not like to wait for their turn
- is restless
- talks excessively and interrupts others

Based upon the diagnostic criteria and this list, it means that students with visual problems can be mistakenly diagnosed with ADD/ADHD. This type of wrong diagnosis happens more often than you think. Lets take a look at some of the facts.

In 2005 David Granet, MD, Professor of Ophthalmology and Pediatrics and Director of the Divisions of Pediatric Ophthalmology and Eye Alignment Disorders at the University of California, San Diego, studied over 266 people who had been diagnosed with CI. Ten percent of these patients were also diagnosed as having ADD and ADHD. This finding, according to Granet and his research team, was three times the number of ADD and ADHD found in the general population. (Granet et al. 2005)

Developmental optometrists, general optometrists, as well as ophthalmologists alike, feel that the overall lack of familiarity with children's vision problems is partially to blame. Excessive attention in the media and in mainstream public opinion on ADD and ADHD merely adds fuel to the fire of misdirected and impatient diagnoses, often determined by the wrong people.

As early as 1970, attention deficit syndromes were considered controversial. Today the controversies range from differing opinions over diagnosis as well as treatment. Perhaps the biggest controversy is over the widespread writing of prescription medication for stimulants when the diagnosis to justify the medication, did not include a comprehensive examination of visual development. In fact, most studies that are performed on children with ADD/ADHD are performed on a child patient population that already has a history of stimulant medication. (Leo, Cohen 2003)

Simply put, prior to any discussion of a child and possible ADD/ADHD, did someone check to see if this child is trying to read with double vision? The author of this book is concerned that too often ADD and ADHD are used as an explanation for behavior in the classroom that is really rooted in the frustration students feel when they are intelligent kids, who want to do well, but are chronically juggling headaches, failure, frustration and anger because they have a binocular dysfunction. They try their hardest, but cannot concentrate. They are compared to other students and siblings and start to loose self-esteem and confidence. Parents and teachers talk about them as learning disabled or disruptive to others at home and at school. All of this because no one took the time to adequately check their binocular vision and whether or not they are being expected to read, when they cannot see the words on the pages at school. Also worth noting is that there should be an evaluation of level of concentration since visual interference makes it difficult to sustain concentration for any length of time.

As a "syndrome" attention deficit disorders are considered to be groupings of symptoms that together characterize either a disease condition or a psychological abnormality.

Any health pattern referred to as a syndrome usually has clusters or patterns of symptoms. Attention disorders are considered to be cognitive disorders and as such may mimic other health problems and vice versa. When symptoms that cannot be objectively measured overlap with other conditions with similar symptoms, it becomes difficult to accurately tease apart one abnormality from another. Worse yet, a person may even have multiple syndromes that intertwine making more than one correct diagnosis necessary in order to get the root of a problem.

ADD and ADHD are misdiagnosed at a rate of four incorrect to every one child who is correctly identified. How can this be? Well, let's look at some of the facts. The Centers for Disease Control and Prevention have published research that has shown that 3 to 7% of school aged children suffer from ADD/ADHD. If we can use 5% as the average, then in a classroom of 25 students only one child will have ADD or ADHD. Yet six or seven or more children are on medication for ADD or ADHD. The drugs they may be taking include: Ritalin and Concerta to name two.

Major publications such as *TIME Magazine, The New York Times, USA Today* and *The Philadelphia Inquirer* have all published articles, which have questioned how these patterns of diagnosis, and drug use can exist.

That pattern of misuse aside, it has also been reported that there have already been quite a few documented deaths attributed to use of these drugs. This suggests that such stimulant drugs might increase the risks of stroke and serious arrhythmias in children and adults. As a result, the Food and Drug Administration (FDA) (a US Federal agency) voted to suggest that these drugs carry the most serious of the agency's drug risk warnings known as a "black box warning." Dr. Steven Nissen, a cardiologist at the Cleveland Clinic and a panel member stated, "I must say that I have grave concerns about the use of these drugs and grave concerns about the harm they may cause."

Many believe that Ritalin is addictive. Bruce Wiseman, National President of the Citizen's Commission on Human Rights (CCHR is a psychiatric watchdog group), notes that the US Drug Enforcement Agency has labeled Ritalin as a class 1 narcotic, sharing the spotlight with morphine, opium and cocaine. Be aware, these are NOT mild drugs. Drugs in this class have potential and significant side effects and they are not the same as giving your child long term antibiotics for acne or cough medicine for a cold.

Again, we ask, how can this be? Here is a common and frequently occurring scenario: A teacher or counselor at school tells a parent that their child is fidgety at school and appears to be unable to concentrate for very long. They recommend the parents to take the child to a doctor to get some medication that will help. Mom or Dad takes their son or daughter to see a doctor as suggested and re-state to the physician the recommendation from the teacher. They report that the teacher has noticed that their child lacks in skills need to be able to concentrate. The physician usually responds with a written prescription, commenting that it should help the child concentrate better and condones the teacher's request.

Questions should already be in your mind about how accurate the intent of the treatment (albeit a prescription drug) matches the diagnosis of the problem for this child. This may very well be one of the few areas of healthcare where an invasive intervention is prescribed WITHOUT any objective evaluation or scientifically based measurement of the hypothesis of the diagnosis. Indeed, many feel that children who are treated this way are not given quality access to health care and that the doctor or teacher who holds the hammer sees every child with a concentration problem as a nail. There is a fast growing concern that children's lifestyle issues in our age of technology are being glossed over with impatient quick fixes, inattention and misguided outcomes. Moreover, mothers pick up that something is not right with their child, but are less and less willing to accept the quick-fix prescription solution.

Symptoms of ADD/ADHD are often the same symptoms that occur in other conditions, for example, in binocular dysfunctions or the conditions where the two eyes do not work as a team causing concentration tasks to become difficult and frustrating, not to mention laborious. The best known of the binocular dysfunctions is convergence insufficiency. Actually, a recent study performed under the direction of the National Institutes of Health (NIH) showed that these very symptoms that occur in either ADD or CI (convergence insufficiency) could be eliminated through the use of a noninvasive intervention technique known as vision therapy.

According to a summary of clinical trials published by the American Medical Association, an NIH study on convergence insufficiency proves that CI can cause headaches, double vision, blurry vision, frustration and difficulty concentrating, when expected to do close work and that CI is not an uncommon problem. (Convergence Insufficiency Treatment Trial (CITT) Study Group)

It is important to know that a person can have CI and still do very well on a standard eye exam that tests for 20/20 eyesight in each individual eye. *20/20 is not enough.* Please understand that an eye exam by many eye doctors very well may not uncover convergence insufficiency because it has not been tested for. Countless studies confirm that CI interferes with reading because it interferes with the ability to see. CI further manifests itself in the lack of ability to learn up to your potential because of the inability to work well at a close distance such as the close work required in school, particularly for reading.

Once again referring to the study completed by the National Eye Institute and reprinted by the American Medical Association proves that office-based vision therapy is the most successful treatment for CI. Home based therapy, often referred to as "pencil pushup therapy" was shown in studies to be ineffective for the treatment of CI. (Convergence Insufficiency Treatment Trial (CITT) Study Group)

Again, vision therapy is not a panacea. Vision therapy helps improve reading or solve school problems because it provides students with the vision needed to better concentrate and engage in reading as an activity. Vision therapy enables the mind to concentrate while reading and thus, learn from what is read. Vision therapy does not treat addiction, but may help to prevent one by allowing a student to feel connected to others and grounded in the world, often referred to as "healthy human attachment."

There continues to also be a concern that developmental and cultural differences in children may also fuel widespread careless diagnoses of ADD and ADHD. Other studies conclude that ADD and ADHD may also be mistaken for developmental differences between children and that often "normal" child behavior is forgotten in favor of medicalization of behavior. Often it is the younger children in a grade that are thought to have ADD and ADHD. One cannot help but wonder what influences parenting style has on a child's behavior as well as influences that may be rooted in the health of the home environment.

Let's take a moment now and look at a case study. Phillip was only in first grade when school problems started to surface. By second grade he was falling further behind and no one could figure out why. His IQ scores were in the 98th percentile and a standard eye examination had revealed a mild case of farsightedness so he was given glasses to "correct" the condition.

Still he reversed letters and numbers, skipped and/or reread words, couldn't concentrate, his mind wandered and he became frustrated and angry during reading group. He made no improvement even working with a reading tutor. The school psychologist determined that he was suffering from an "incipient learning disability." Phillip's case is not unique. It happens frequently.

While traditional eye care has advanced significantly in the areas of pathology and surgery, the regular eye exam is, in many ways, stuck in the early 1900s. In fact the Snellen chart, used to measure 20/20 eyesight was invented during the Civil War. Many people have the idea that certain learning disabilities will be outgrown. The research tells us that 73% of all children with reading/learning disorders have binocular and/or perceptual dysfunctions. Most parents believe if their child has 20/20 eyesight, it is perfect. *Not true.*

The difference between sight and vision are crucial to the understanding of ADD/ ADHD, reading and learning disabilities, and autism. Sight occurs in the eyes: and, vision occurs in the brain. Since vision is our dominant sense (80% of learning occurs thru the visual sense), the importance of that interplay between eyes and brain is critical. If children begin to fall behind, it can affect their self-confidence and affect the rest of their lives. Many will develop the " I can't do it " syndrome. This is a sort of "learned helplessness" where the child becomes accustom to failure, and thinks of himself as unable to achieve and learn.

The symptoms of binocular dysfunctions include: can't concentrate, mind wanders, short attention span, easily distractible, etc. Sounds like ADD/ADHD, doesn't it? This is why so many kids are misdiagnosed with ADD/ADHD and placed on drugs. Many parents are frustrated because no one can tell them why. So it is easy to accept medication as the answer. But when non-scientific criteria are used to label normal childhood behavior or misdiagnosed conditions, the problem of ADD/ ADHD reflects a problem with adults and not a problem with the children and this has become an epidemic.

When adults gloss over symptoms observed in children, or fail to correctly diagnose and refer, it becomes a problem with shortcomings in adults. Worse yet, when adults recommend, prescribe and administer drugs from the amphetamine class to children, in place of accurate diagnosis or problem solving, this epidemic becomes widespread social neglect.

Woven within the epidemic of ADD/ADHD (which coincides with the increase in pharmaceutical marketing practices) is one of the major problems of health in the United States: unnoticed poor vision. Symptoms of poor vision often go unrecognized because what is noticed instead, are its consequences which are more observable. The consequences to a child learning to read with poor vision are decreased learning ability, lower self esteem, poor self-concept, emotional imbalance and failure to learn to read and keep up with the other kids. Teachers often label vision related manifestations as "a learning disability." It is then a short diving board from the phrase "learning disability" to "I think your child has ADHD." From the "ADHD" label, the slippery slope includes drug induced behavior modification.

Students are often labeled as seeking attention, having poor concentration skills or as disruptive to the class when in fact they are having vision problems. Vision problems in young children are common because the visual system is still developing. Visual problems have a direct influence on behavior even if it is as simple as liking or disliking school and or homework.

Dr. Seiderman's research, published in 1980 on a child population labeled as have learning disability, found that 73% of those thought to be learning disabled also had binocular and or perceptual visual problems that were correctable. (Seiderman 1980) Hokoda confirmed as well that 21% of the general childhood population had binocular visual problems that are treatable. (Hokoda 1985)

So far, in this chapter, the reader should be picking up several deep rooted frustrations with the American health care industry and the American educational system. Lets review some of the facts again:

- Vision problems that influence a child's ability to do well in school are going unrecognized and undertreated at an alarming rate. Why?

- Why are pediatricians, ophthalmologists and psychiatrists continuing to ignore the neurological, perceptual and intellectual components of healthy vision in favor of surgery or prescription drugs? So often, when convergence insufficiency (CI) is diagnosed, there is avoidance in referring the patient to a behavioral optometrist for evaluation for vision therapy. At a minimum, why aren't patients informed that CI can be treated without surgery or drugs, by a behavioral optometrist? Again, lack of this information to the patient hinders the opportunity for informed consent on the patient's behalf.

- Many children with untreated visual perceptual problems are instead told they have ADD/ADHD. They are socialized as having a "learning disability" and this severely affects their self esteem and confidence.

- Normal kid behavior has become medicalized. The labeling is carelessly applied and omits the consideration of other important diagnostic tests to identify real physiological problems such as convergence insufficiency.

- Lack of attention in school and at home can be due to a number of other problems unrelated to ADD/ADHD.

- Children in our school systems are being drugged by parents, teachers and physicians, in order to modify behavior. The drugs most commonly used are in the amphetamine class, similar to cocaine, carry a black box warning and are addictive. When tolerance to the drug is observed, the dosage is usually increased.

- The number of deaths due to side effects, drug toxicity as well as teenage suicide attempts is rising as these drugs are made more readily available and adults become more dependent upon them to manage the youth of today.

- Marketing of drugs earmarked as ADD/ADHD treatments form children has increased exponentially. The massive amount of marketing and advertising has resulted in increased sales and prescribing of these drugs. In fact over the last 30 years the *Diagnostic and Statistical Manual of Mental Disorders (DSM IV)* criteria for attention disorders has relaxed the language for the diagnostic criteria allowing for greater inclusion in insurance coverage. Many feel this fuels the prescription writing.

- Let's not forget that there is no valid objective test for ADD/ADHD.

- Generally speaking, pediatricians, ophthalmologists and general optometrists still use the 20/20 eye chart, also known as the "Snellen Chart" as the benchmark for acceptable vision, but the 20/20 Snellen test is not enough to check for the health of "total vision." Vision that feeds the brain with sensory material that the brain needs in order to make sense of input from the visual world.

The false sense of a "thorough vision exam" by only relying upon the 20/20 Snellen test misleads parents and the public into believing that a complete vision exam has been performed, when in fact, the child has only had an "eye exam" and not a full vision examination.

In Phillip's case, like many other children, he was unable to make his eyes work together as a team (CI). Phillip was unable to get the two images from his two eyes to fuse into one. He reported seeing double at a distance of 10 inches from his nose. Imagine trying to concentrate on reading or homework while seeing double. Phillip began a noninvasive program of vision therapy. After about 20 sessions, Phillip was reading at grade level and his schoolwork improved dramatically, allowing him to fulfill his intellectual potential. We see a significant improvement with about 90% of these patients. Parents report vast improvements in concentration, reading, and learning along with a healthy increase in self-confidence.

Phillip, from the case study just presented, went on to attend and graduate from an Ivy League college. Today he is successful, confident, and above all else, a happy and well adjusted adult.

Again, it cannot be overemphasized that the 20/20 Snellen Chart (the chart that checks each eye individually to see how far you can focus and read letters on the wall) does not constitute a vision examination. Vision requires each eye to work together as a team so that you have good depth perception, peripheral vision and fuse together that which each eye sees independently. In addition, the processing of visual information is critical. Total vision is needed for the brain to function properly.

Having healthy functioning vision allows us to have healthy interaction with our environment and the people in it. When our total vision is healthy, we comprehend better, we think better and our brain functions at its best. We can focus better, learn better and maximize that which our intellect allows. Simply put, when our vision is optimal, we do better cognitively. Vision refers to our ability to understand what we see and develop the intellect.

REFERENCES

Granet DB, Gomi CF, Ventura R, Miller-Scholte A 2005. The relationship between convergenc insufficiency and ADHD. Strabismus 13:163-68.

Leo, Cohen 2003. Broken brains or flawed studies? A critical review of ADHD Neuroimaging studies. J Mind Behavior 24:29-56.

Convergence Insufficiency Treatment Trial (CITT) Study Group. A Randomized Clinical Trial of Convergence Insufficiency in Children. American Medical Association Reprint from Arch Opthalmol 2005;123.

Seiderman AS 1980. Optometric vision therapy results of a demonstration project with a learning disabled population. J Am Optom Assoc 51:489-93.

Hokoda SC 1985. General binocular dysfunctions in an urban optometry clinic. J Am Optom Assoc 56:560-62.

RECOMMENDED READING

Attention Deficit Hyperactivity Disorder www.nimh.nih.gov U.S. Dept of Health and Human Services. National Institute of Health, NIH Publication No. 08-3572 Revised 2008.

Cooper J, Cooper R. Conditions Associated with Strabismus: Convergence Insufficiency. Optometrists Network, All About Strabismus. 2001-2005.

Bartiss M. Extraocular Muscles: Convergence Insufficiency. eMedicine.com, Inc., eMedicine Specialties, Ophthalmology. 2005.

Birnbaum MH, Soden R, Cohen AH. Efficacy of vision therapy for convergence insufficiency in an adult male population. J Am Optom Assoc. 1999;70:225-32.

Dehaene S. Reading in the Brain. New York: Viking, 2009.

Eide B, Eide F. The Mislabeled Child. New York: Hyperion, 2006.

Farrar R, Call M, Maples WC. A comparison of the visual symptoms between ADD/ADHD and normal children. Optometry 2001;72:441-51.

Kranowitz CS. The Out-of-Sync Child. New York: Penguin Group, 1998.

Orfield A. Eyes for Learning. Lanham, Maryland: Rowman & Littlefield Education, 2007

Rouse MW, Borsting E, Hyman L, Hussein M, Cotter SA, Flynn M, Scheiman M, Gallaway M, De Land PN. Frequency of convergence insufficiency among fifth and sixth graders. Optom Vis Sci. 1999;76:643-49.

Scheiman M, Mitchell GL, Cotter S, et al; the Convergence Insufficiency Treatment Trial (CITT) Study Group. A randomized clinical trial of treatments for convergence insufficiency in children. Archives of Ophthalmology. 2005;123:14-24. Complete article - PDF version.

Scheiman M, Cooper J, Mitchell GL, et al. A survey of treatment modalities for convergence insufficiency. Optom Vis Sci. 2002;79:151-57.

Seiderman AS. Optometric vision therapy -- results of a demonstration project with a learning disabled population. J Am Optom Assoc. 1980;51:489-93.

Convergence Insufficiency Treatment Trial Study Group. Randomized clinical trial of treatments for symptomatic convergence insufficiency in children. Archives of Ophthalmology. 2008;126:1336-49.

Edmund JS Sonuga-Brke, Sarah Elgie, Martin Hall. *More to ADHA than Meets the Eye; observable abnormalities in search behavior do not account for performance deficits on a discrimination task.* Behavior and Brain Functions 2005;1:10.

Solan HA, Shelley-Tremblay JF, Hansen PC, Larson S. *Is there a common linkage among reading comprehension, visual attention, and magnocellular processing?* J Learn Disabil 2007;40:270-78.

Solan HA, Shelley-Tremblay J, Larson S. *Vestibular function, sensory integration, and cognitive and balance abnormalities: a brief literature review.* J Optom Vis Dev 2007;38:1-5.

O'Brien N, Langhinrichsen-Rohling J, Shelley-Tremblay JF. *Reading problems, Attentional deficits, and current mental health problems in adjudicated adolescent males.* J Correct Edu 2007;58:3.

Solan HA, Shelley-Tremblay J, Larson S, Mounts J. *Silent word reading fluency and temporal vision processing: differences between good and poor readers.* J Behav Optom 2006;17:1-9.

Solan HA, Shelley-Tremblay J, Hansen P, Larson S, Ficarra AP. *M-Cell Deficits and reading disability: A preliminary study on the effects of temporal vision processing therapy.* optometry, Optometry 2004 Oct;75:640-50.

Solan H.A., Shelley-Tremblay J, Larson S. *Effect of attention therapy on reading comprehension.* J Learn Disabil 2003;36:556-63.

Solan HA, Larson S, Shelley-Tremblay JF, Silverman M, Ficarra AP. *The role of visual attention in cognitive control of oculomotor readiness in learning disabled 6th graders.* J Learn Disabil 2001;34:107-18.

Shelley-Tremblay JF, Rosen LA. *Attention Deficit Hyperactivity Disorder: An Evolutionary Perspective.* J Genet Psychol 1996;157:443-53.

Waber DP. *Rethinking Learning Disabilities.* New York: Guilford Press, 2010.

CHAPTER 6
VISION, DRUG USE AND
ALTERING PERCEPTION

We hope none of the readers of this book can relate to this chapter on the topic of addiction and addictive behavior. In truth, we know this hope is not real. Studies show that over 9% percent of Americans aged 12 and above have a serious substance abuse problem. (*Washington Times*, September 6, 2003) Of this group, certain percentages are young adults and children. Never before have recreational and illicit use of prescription drugs been so available to kids. Never before have so many teen idols erroneously socialized our youth with the notion that it is not so bad to get caught using drugs. Never before have our youth gotten so easily pardoned, from a social standpoint, after drug rehab, only to fall prey to repeated patterns of past behaviors.

Addictive behavior shows no partiality to age, race, social status, gender or intellect. In fact, when we think about it, we are all addicted to something. While you may like to exercise, I may like to eat chocolate. We do these activities repetitively and mindlessly. Why? Because they make us feel good. If you ask a thumb sucking kid why they suck their thumb, you will most likely hear them say, "Because it feels good." It is also likely that you are hard pressed to get them to stop. So, too, is the case with prescription and street drug abuse.

While the majority of people turn to food, alcohol, gambling or cruising the Internet, others turn to drugs. In the chapter on ADD/ADHD we talked about prescription drugs being given to many children who actually have binocular vision problems such as convergence insufficiency with symptoms that overlap with those of ADD/ADHD. In this chapter we cover the same binocular visual concerns, but in children who end up getting their prescription for relief from the street.

So what does addiction or drug use have to do with vision? Well, we're glad you asked and are curious enough to still be with us in reading this chapter. Since a certain percentage of people in our society become addicted to drugs and another percentage have vision problems, it makes sense that there are a proportion of people who share both problems.

Does one cause the other? Does addiction presuppose a vision problem? Does a vision problem, such as convergence insufficiency or difficulty with perception or environment interpretation, presuppose addictive behavior? Who knows! It is not the goal of this chapter to prove or statistically demonstrate any cause effect relationship.

What we do know is that people who fall prey to substance abuse to get through their day, are confused individuals. They are confused because they need to escape reality. They are confused because they are getting negative feedback from their environment. They are particularly confused because they "don't fit in" When they finally do feel like they fit in, it is only when they are "high" on their "drug of choice."

Some drugs actually alter visual perception. Some drugs alter depth of vision, and others affect ability to focus and track accurately. Do the visual changes provide relief? Do the visual changes give their brains a rest from other visual chaos and confusion? None of these questions can be answered for certain without the funding necessary for clinical trials and scientific study. What we do know is that there are plenty of families who struggle to make sense of the craziness that accompanies addiction. Every one of those families eventually "waits for the phone call." They all hope it is a call from the addict, ready to resign their old behavior in favor of a willingness to accept help. More often than not it is a call from someone else, with the inevitably dreaded news.

Most importantly, we know that an addiction is the compulsive need for something, whether substance or pattern of activity, that is needed for survival. The critical piece here is that these substances or activities never truly satisfy the addict. They do not fully satisfy because they do not deal with the real problem. A drug addict does not really need drugs to get through their day but they do need something. If that need is not accurately identified, the confused individual may perceive drugs to be the answer.

In some cases the root of the problem may be an undiagnosed binocular or visual processing problem. They may have a common condition called convergence insufficiency (CI) and they may actually be in need of professional help with vision.

Convergence insufficiency is more common than many parents may realize. When a child or adult is struggling with the consequence of untreated convergence insufficiency, they are experiencing an inability to maintain binocular vision. Proper binocular vision requires the eyes to maintain alignment on objects as they approach from distance to close range.

Symptoms associated with CI vary from mild to severe, and are extremely troublesome for those patients with this condition. Unconsciously and consciously, the person suffering with convergence insufficiency desperately tries to get through their day. They are operating in survival mode rather than as a thriving individual. This affects their stamina, their self-esteem, their successes and failures as well as their choice of friends. They don't fit in, no matter how hard they try. Often, others who "don't fit in" become comfortable companions to hang around with. In short, they are vulnerable individuals and are easy prey for the street drug industry.

By now you may understand that the addict, as a vulnerable individual, may need help with how they see the world in which they live. It is for all the reasons above that we have included this chapter in this book on vision therapy. The addict may need help from a behavioral optometrist and vision therapy may help them with a means to get off and stay off of drugs, or actually prevent them from becoming addicted.

When kids are having a hard time coping with life's ordinary demands, drugs sometimes seem to make life easier. Unfortunately, youth in our society are exposed to drugs at a rate never before in history. The child quietly struggling with double vision or lack of concentration that is interfering with success in school may indeed have the same problems as the ADD/ADHD appearing student.

The quiet student, perhaps shy and less outgoing, who does not disrupt the family or make a fuss in class, may just turn their frustration inward rather than outward. With the rate of Ritalin buying and selling, trading and crushing to share and snort together in school, as high as it is, what would stop a struggling student from trying something that seemed to be helping the other kids? After all, we live in a society that has socialized adults and children that solutions to life's problems can be fast and easy. Just take a pill. Little do they realize the price paid when they choose this option.

While binocular visual problems may be misidentified as ADD/ADHD, at least someone, somewhere along the way, notices that something is wrong with a child. Other kids, often those who are very bright, try to manage on their own. As they meet each daily challenge with greater and greater difficulty and desiring to "fit in" with everyone else, they become vulnerable to anything that gives them relief or an escape. Simply put, life can be hard, and drugs can be easy.

Most of the chapters in the book, compile proven facts from years worth of experience and published literature. This chapter is different. We are not turning to written works on drugs, we are writing from the heart. We are not here to prove a point or imply a "magic bullet." This chapter is written at the frontier of vision science, and brings you only anecdotal evidence. Parents dealing with drug addicted kids are foremost in our thoughts. Meanwhile we hope that we help the drug addicted person as well. Most of all, this chapter is written with kindness, care and the hope for healing.

The literature tells us that drug and/or alcohol addiction is inherited. We also understand that there is no "cure." For the sake of our discussion, we will use five years "clean" as a cure rate, albeit, advisedly so. The question, then, becomes, why is the "cure rate" less than 12%. One has a better chance of recovering from most cancers than drug addiction. When the addict enters a drug rehab program for six weeks or six months, or whatever, what services are provided? Does the individual receive individual psychological counseling to determine what set of circumstances or underlying problems pushed the person to drug usage? Many, if not most, are bipolar. Has this been addressed with the correct medications, and have the medications been adjusted properly? Has vocational instruction, guidance, and job placement been handled? Many if not most, have huge concentration difficulties. Of course, that is where binocular vision and perceptual skill development comes into play. If all of the aforementioned is not addressed, then the addict is ultimately released " clean." However, he or she is released from the rehab program "clean" of drugs; but he or she must face the exact same environment in which he failed previously. Why would we not expect a relapse in drug addiction?

Vision problems signal that something inside the brain is out of balance, but this is not easy to pick up if you think that everyone sees what you see. If you find out you have a vision problem and have it treated with vision therapy, not only is your vision improved, but so too is your insight and your cognitive skills. This in turn, allows you to have a better outlook on life, to problem solve and visualize better solutions to problems and this in turn helps foster better vision all around. In fact, you see yourself in a better way. Many, if not most, addicts have poor problem solving skills. Poor problem solving skills lead to poor decision making.

Now imagine that you have a visual perception problem. No one seems to notice that you have problems or that something is not quite right. You yourself do not know you have visual perceptual problems, and you have no idea that you need help. You manage to fall through every crack in the system, and you are out there problem solving life on your own.

It is unlikely that you have a good view of yourself or your place in the world, and you may actually feel quite disconnected. You feel like a misfit, a square peg trying to fit into a round hole. You find that drugs alter your perception. You get relief. In fact, using drugs helps to hide your problems. Now you seem to fit right in.

Some of the most common street drugs include cocaine, crack-cocaine, metham-phetamine, marijuana, Ritalin, steroids, LSD, ecstasy, inhalants and heroin. Here are some facts about some of these drugs with emphasis on effects on the visual perceptual and visual systems.

In general hallucinogens like heroin, LSD, cocaine and marijuana alter the senses. They effect changes in the visual, auditory and tactile senses, but mostly affect visual perception. Hallucinatory drugs will allow a user to experience sharper distinctions of color as well as alter the ability to concentrate. People addicted to hallucinogens can often visualize things like geometric shapes without closing their eyes. They may also experience the cross referencing of senses in ways that allows them to see sounds and hear visual items. In general, colors are brighter and objects are sharper.

Meanwhile, drugs in the amphetamine class are stimulants producing increased wakefulness and increased focus. Ritalin, Adderall and the other drugs used to treat ADD/ADHD are performance enhancers, which fall into this class. These drugs have the potential for both addiction as well as abuse. On the street, Ritalin may be referred to as 'uppers" or "beanies" among other names, and they do produce a "high." They increase energy, attention and focus. Same thing with Adderall, which produces a feeling of well being, increased concentration and focus, and improves study skills.

Right here is a good place to share with you, the reader, why this chapter has been written and included in this book. Dr. Seiderman possesses no special knowledge or formal study in drug addiction. His experience with this topic is first hand from observation within his extended family. As such, assertions made in this chapter are based upon direct observation and personal experience.

The author noticed that an adult family member who went through rehab repeatedly continues to struggle to overcome addiction. He lived with his parents for a couple of years off and on when he was clean. He worked hard and had a good job during that time. Then one day he vanished. He saved everything, then one day he was nowhere to be found and on a "run." During the time that he lived back home, he brought numerous friends to the home with him. Dr. Seiderman took note that they all had a similar quality, and that none of them could concentrate. It seemed that each had an early pattern of experience with repeated failure, although possessing exceptional intelligence, which led to exhaustive frustration and the "feeling" that they simply did not "fit in."

Given his lifelong experience with patterns of behavior associated with vision problems, he noticed specific behaviors that raised all sorts of questions related to the ability to concentrate. Again, the point of this chapter is not to make the statement that vision therapy can cure drug dependency. Perhaps though, visual disturbances might be a contributing factor that is being terribly overlooked.

One can only imagine what goes through the mind of a kid in 8th grade who can't concentrate, and just simply cannot achieve no matter how hard he tries. They have trouble maintaining good grades and may not even be able to finish school. The bottom line is that they start to feel like they just do not fit into society. They cannot meet the expectations of academic or social environments. They don't fit in with the geeky kids. They don't fit in with the athletic kids. They don't seem to fit in with anyone except with their friends who use drugs. School and society are hard, and drugs are easy. Quoting the family member, "When I am on my drug of choice, I feel like I fit in." The important thing to be mindful of here is that, this is how they feel, in spite of the fact that others do not perceive them as anything other than potential for success, and very intelligent. Others would see them as "fitting in" but they do not feel that way, except when they are using their "drug of choice." It seems that the downward spiral of addiction is triggered by a drive to be free from "failure" and to find a place where they feel they "belong." Again, this short chapter in a book on binocular visual problems is not an end all and be all or an answer to drug problems in our schools. We are not suggesting any final answers. It is just that perhaps for some of the people struggling to make sense of addictive patterns of behavior, it may be an answer. For these people, there could very well be an unidentified visual component.

It is important to know how addictive the prescription drugs used to treat ADD and ADHD are. It is also important to understand the fine line between access to them through a prescription versus getting them on the street or trading in the schools. It happens, and it happens more often than parents realize.

At a minimum, prescription use of Ritalin or Adderall can lead a young person down the road to try other drugs, try drugs off the street and pave the path for addictions of other kinds. Undiagnosed vision problems, misidentified, as ADD/ADHD with prescription drugs to manage the child can be a short journey to street drugs. Parents, please consider a complete visual evaluation by a qualified vision therapy fellow if your child has unexplained behavior that leads you to suspect drug use, or if you are told your child needs medication for ADD/ADHD and you are skeptical of the diagnosis.

It is estimated that 12% of high school students admitted to trying Ritalin at least once without getting it by prescription. Interviewers who talked with students about their experiences with Ritalin additionally expressed concern of health professionals about the over diagnosis of ADD/ADHD and the misuse of the drugs to treat it. Many are particularly concerned about Ritalin overprescribing.

In June 2001, *CBS News Health Watch* reported that at a Rhode Island Middle School, sixth graders were charged with possessing and distributing drugs, while a similar situation was simultaneously discovered at a school in Florida. Students admitted to using the behavior altering drug, Ritalin in order "to fit in," to "get up in the morning," "to get their school work done" or just "to be cool." On *CBS News* Terry Woodworth of the US Drug Enforcement Administration (DEA) likened Ritalin to "Kiddie Cocaine." (www.cbsnews.com/stories/2002/01/31/health/main327150.shtml)

The report went on to further say that many teenagers think it is cool to use an illicit drug that other students get legally from their parents or from the school nurse. Of these drugs Ritalin is the most popular. Woodworth claims that this is a significant problem in the US.

The report went on to also say that with 11 million prescriptions for Ritalin given out every year, kids get the impression that Ritalin is safe, not to mention easy to get. Students who are prescribed the drug go on to sell it for a few dollars a pill. A public health study completed on 3,500 students in Massachusetts found that 12.7% admitted to using Ritalin that was prescribed to another student.

In the CBS news report a young man (age 18) from a Boston suburb recalls his story. He was prescribed Ritalin as a child, but started selling his pills in the seventh grade. "I also started snorting it at that time," he said. "Other kids were doing it and it gave you a little bit of a buzz, and allowed you to stay up a little longer."

Although he's now clean, he is convinced that abusing Ritalin set him on an even more dangerous course. "I ended up doing a lot of stronger amphetamines that brought me down pretty quick, and I don't know if I would have gotten interested in them if I hadn't started using Ritalin." In summary, if you think your child has turned to drugs, here are some recommendations:

- Do not try to solve their problem.

- Do not tell them what to do.

- Do not criticize them.

- Do not shut them out.

- Do not deprive them of your love.

- Do not ignore them.

- Most of all, do not take on more than you can handle.

- Do seek outside help.

- Do consider a complete visual examination by a qualified behavioral optometrist.

- Do not settle for a basic eye exam that measures ability to focus only with each individual eye as measured by the 20/20 Snellen chart.

- Do seek psychological counselling, preferably by a psychologist experienced in dependency problems.

- Do encourage participation in local anonymous addiction programs, such as AA (Alcoholics Anonymous) or NA (Narcotics Anonymous).

REFERENCE

The Washington Times September 6, 2003 "22 Million Americans are Addicts" http://www.washtimes.com/national/20030906-120039-1281r.htm

www.cbsnews.com/stories/2002/01/31/health/main327150.shtml

RECOMMENDED READING

Johnston, L.D., O'Malley, P.M. & Bachman, J.G. (2001) Monitoring the Future: National Survey Results on Drug Use, 1975-2000. Volume 1: Secondary School Students (NIH Publication No. 01-4924), Bethesda, MD: National Institute on Drug Abuse.

CHAPTER 7
AUTISM AND ASPERGER'S SYNDROME

The mind is an amazing part of the human spirit, influencing how we view our personhood in the world and what we make of the opportunities in life. What is reality? Does anyone of us know that answer? Is there an answer? Realistically, none of us has the exact same level of patience, learning capacity or resilience from day to day. Some of us are morning people, others perform well at night. We cannot think as well when we are tired or overloaded and most people can relate to fluctuations in performance ability, often referred to as "a spectrum."

Autism, Asperger syndrome, executive function ability, ADD and ADHD are often thought of as a spectrum of disorders (ASD), understood on a continuum that fluctuates from day to day and with levels of stress. Some of these terms are associated with what is often referred to as a "learning disability." The author of this book, prefers not to think in terms of learning disability, but rather to help readers understand that not everyone sees the world the same way. Our brain plasticity and cognitive ability are directly related to what the senses deliver to the brain and how the world is conceptualized according to sensory input. In the case of visual input and cognitive processing of this input, the eyes account for at least 80% input, leaving, sound, taste and touch with the remainder.

So this begs the questions... What really is a learning disability? Are learning disabilities simple enough to define and categorize? Is there such a thing as a learning disability or are they merely variations on ways of navigating in the world? Can the acquisition of knowledge be standardized in a way that includes or excludes variations in learning style between what is considered to be normal and that which is in the minority?

Learning variations are very complex and so, too, are their diagnoses. Often, there is more than one type of learning style or learning challenge, so it is important that each case be reviewed individually with specific recommendations in mind.

"I know that all children are different, but..." How many times have you heard that statement? "I know that I shouldn't compare Johnny to Billy, but..." The truth of the matter is that most parents just pay "lip service" to that important concept. They understand, but they don't understand!

Perhaps, the autism spectrum is the great teacher for all of us. The HBO movie, *Temple Grandin,* starring Claire Danes, is a must see for all readers of this book and particularly of this chapter. This award winning documentary-turned-movie is not just for autistic individuals and their parents.

Why is this movie so important? Because it demonstrates how we are all different. Granted, the behaviors of the autistic individual are more exaggerated than most, but if you understand those differences, the application to parenting and working with children becomes clearer. The movie shows how a mother, aunt, and science teacher enable Temple Grandin (an autistic child) to learn, and channel her strengths into an extraordinary success story.

The picture painted is of a young woman's perseverance and struggle with autism at a time when it was relatively unknown (1960s). Again, to re-emphasize, this movie is a must see for all parents and is critical for parents, teachers and families of autistic children. Why is it also important for parents of non-autistic children? Good question—it is important because it demonstrates good parenting and teaching skills.

In 2003, Dr. Grandin spoke to the College of Optometrists in Vision Development (COVD), the professional organization of vision therapists and behavioral optometrists) about vision problems experienced by those with autism. Her meeting with vision therapists at that conference was so inspiring for her that three years later, in 2006, she wrote and Vintage Books published an expanded, second edition of her classic book, *Thinking in Pictures: My Life with Autism.*

Dr. Grandin writes: "If visual processing problems are suspected, the child should see a developmental optometrist. This is a special eye doctor who can do therapy and exercises to help the processing problems that are inside the brain. In many of these children, the eye itself is normal but faulty wiring in the brain is causing the problem."

With all the credit in the world given to the courage and success of Dr. Grandin, we highly recommend that readers of this chapter refer to both of Dr. Grandin's books along with watching the movie which documents her experiences. The first book she published is titled, *Emergence: Labeled Autistic,* and is coauthored with Margaret M. Scariano. In this personal story, Temple relays her childhood; she expresses her regrets that many children are "labeled" autistic when perhaps they are not. She feels that the term has become 'fashionable" and that unfortunately many children, like herself, are given messages that they are low achievers, when in fact they simply function, learn and interact differently. Anyone attempting to better understand autism would be wise to read Temple Grandin's own account of her life with autism.

Parenting is, in Dr. Seiderman's opinion, the second most difficult task we face in our lifetime. Yet, there is no course in our schooling that addresses this task. We are, all, on our own. Most of us take parenting for granted. We assume we know how to be good parents. The movie and Temple Grandin's life experience shows us how this can be accomplished. And, if you give it some thought, it shows how it can be transferred to all children. Maybe a second viewing of the film is in order. Or, possibly, a group viewing with several sets of parents, followed by a discussion of the movie by those attending. Believe me, it is a worthwhile exercise.

An example of one of the very significant differences in Dr. Grandin's behavior is that she sees things and thinks in pictures. Thus, the titles of two of the books she has written and published are: *The Way I See it* and *Thinking in Pictures*. Grandin states, "The best thing a parent of a newly diagnosed child can do is to watch their child, without preconceived notions and judgments, and learn how the child functions, acts, and reacts to his or her world."

Wouldn't you say that is good advice for *any* parent? Effective teachers and good parents understand that for a child to learn, the teaching style must match the learning style of the student. Different thinking patterns of children with ASD require parents and educators to teach from a new frame of reference, one that matches the child's learning style.

Teachers who expect the autistic child to fit into the traditional social behaviors and lesson plan, only frustrate the child, their classmates and the teacher ultimately fails to see any accomplishment on their own part. Truthfully, doesn't this concept for effective teaching apply to all children? I think so! How we find the child's area is detailed in Grandin's book, *The Way I See It*.

So, what can we all learn from this extraordinary woman and the extraordinary family she had? Further, what can we learn from her exemplary teachers who did not let her down, teachers who looked within themselves to craft a path of success in practicing the art of education for even the most challenging students?

Since we have emphasized the importance of watching this movie, which truly "says it all," let us leave you with one example from the movie of "seeing things differently."

There are numerous scenes where Temple has to walk through a set of sensored sliding glass doors to enter a store. To most people, these are simply glass doors that work automatically and people walk through them to go in and out of a building. In the movie, Temple is afraid of these doors. Why? Because her brain, upon seeing these doors, flips to a visual of a guillotine and she is absolutely petrified, often needing assistance to enter or exit.

When we think about this example, we can each think of a situation in our own lives that allow us to relate to her seemingly irrational fear. When I was a kid, someone threw me into the water, thinking that this method of teaching kids to swim was foolproof. "Throw them in, they'll learn what to do on their own." Well, not so. It created an absolute fear of water for me. As a result, when I am at the beach or near a pool, trusted friends are transformed into traitors in my mind. I see faces ready to knock me off by pushing me in. I do not trust them and these very same cherished friends elicit sheer fear in my eyes and in my mind. Their smiles are not friendly, they are sneering. Their posture is not trustworthy, it is ready for attack.

Anyone who digs deep down introspectively can think of an example of such a phenomenon from his or her own life. Well, imagine for the autistic child. They have more examples of this mental imagery and perhaps a more profound version of it. How can we not help understand their difference as they try, just as we do to navigate each day in their lives?

Overlooked is a book about brain function and efficiency in performance. It is a book that uses brain enhancement activities and vision therapy to teach the mind to work at peak proficiency. The contents of *Overlooked: 20/20 is Not Enough* is no longer on a little known topic.

On September 11, 2007, the *New York Times* ran an article on learning disorders and difficulty with schoolwork when a child's eyes are not working together. The article "Not Autistic or Hyperactive. Just Seeing Double at Times," by Laura Novak, informed the public of behavioral problems that often erupt when a child sees double because their eyes fail to function together at close range even with 20/20 eyesight. An estimated 5% of school children have a condition known as convergence insufficiency and it is most frustrating and painful for these children to learn to read. Often they are labeled as disorderly, hyperactive, even autistic because of how they try to manage headaches, dizziness, nausea, irritability, low self esteem and inability to concentrate, let alone attempt to learn.

Dr. Arthur Seiderman authored one of the first published papers on autism in 1973, a time when autism was not a common household word. Now, unlike then, families either know of, or struggle themselves with a child who has autism or Asperger's syndrome. Dr. Seiderman first came into contact with autism a year earlier, in 1972, while drafting a research paper to fulfill degree requirements for a masters degree in psychology. Dr. Seiderman studied at the Gesell Institute of Child Development at Yale University.

At that time few people had even heard of autism and only a few people had written on the subject. Leo Kanner at Johns Hopkins University was the leader in the field at that time along with Bernard Rimland, Bruno Bettleheim (best known as author of "The Children of the Dream"), Ole Ivar Lovaas and Hans Asperger.

Leo Kanner (1943) and Eugene Bleuler (1911) were among the early users of the term "autism" which originated from the Greek term "autos" or "self" and implied that the self was isolated from social interaction. At one time, autism was considered to be triggered by emotional trauma. With advances in knowledge of autism as a brain development disorder, such an etiological assumption has been corrected. If you are interested in an early documentary on how families with autism were perceived, you may view the film, *Refrigerator Mothers*, at: http://www.snagfilms. com/films/title/refrigerator_mothers (last accessed on 11/7/11)

In the 1940s Dr. Kanner of Johns Hopkins University as well as Hans Asperger of Vienna began to describe the characteristics of what would later be identified as Asperger's syndrome, considered to be a form of high functioning autism. (www.webmd.com/brain/autism/tc/aspergers-syndrome-symptoms)(Last accessed 7/24/12) In the 1960s and 1970s research and treatment for autism was focused on the use of medication, later changing in the 1980s and 1990s to the important role of behavior therapy in managing both autism and Asperger's.

Today we have a better understanding of the autism spectrum disorders, however it has been hard to shake the misconceptions as well as the stigmas associated with developmentally different personality traits.

According to the Mayo Clinic, autism falls under the umbrella category of serious childhood developmental problems called autism spectrum disorders. (www.mayoclinic.com/health/autism) (Last accessed 7/24/12) These spectrum disorders appear in early childhood usually before the age of three and affect a child's ability to communicate and interact with others.

People with autism or Asperger's have difficulty interacting with other people and with the environment around them. It is quite possible that the developing child who has tendencies toward these spectrum disorders develop in ways that manifest an outcome of seeing their environment differently from the majority. Thus, they learn to interpret and understand the world around them from a radically different point of view than those whose minds interpret their life from outside this spectrum of thinking.

Simply put, the life of someone with autism is built upon an alternative foundation for reality. All individuals do this, so this is not to say that there is a hierarchy of reality and that some realities are better than others. No one knows true reality, all we know is that the person with autism subscribes to a different and perhaps minority view of the construction of reality and interpretation of the world and how it works and how, as a result, he or she thinks.

It is important to remember that all autism disorders are not alike and that symptoms and severity can vary greatly. The symptoms tend to fall into three distinct categories and these three areas of concern critically affect the development of a child. The three categories of child development most observed are: social interaction, the child's behavior and language (ability to communicate). Rigid, stereotyped, repetitive patterns of unusual behavior are frequently present. Sleep problems occur in those found to have autism at a rate of between 40% and 70%. (www.aswtcc.org) (Last accessed 7/24/12)

It is important for families to know that scientific studies have proven that parenting style in and of itself is not reflective of whether or not children develop autism and that autism is a multifaceted, multisystem disorder. This is a very important point to repeatedly communicate to those parenting an autistic child.

"Autism" is a term for what authors of *The Diagnostic and Statistical Manual of Mental Disorders*, better known as the DSM-IV criteria, chose to call "PDD" or "Pervasive Developmental Disorder."(American Psychiatric Association 2000)

Since there is technically "no cure" for autism, early preventive and interceptive treatment can make all the difference in the world to a child struggling with this syndrome. Early guidance is equally as important to the rest of the family and parents as well. Early treatment may include psychological counseling for the child. Counseling needs to be available for the parents as well. Parents need to be advised on how to manage and interact with an autistic child as well deal with their child's different and unusual behaviors.

Occupational therapy is usually helpful through the use of sensory integration therapy to reduce tactile defensiveness, along with some physical therapy. A pediatric occupational therapist can also help by integrating communication therapy into the treatment plan. This helps the autistic child to use computer keyboards, letter boards and word boards as a method for auditory integration training. This allows the child to listen to specially prepared sounds through headphones.

Vision therapy is another important interceptive therapeutic phase in helping the child with autism. Vision therapy helps to improve perception and perceptual motor skills along with increasing the child's self esteem and confidence. If we believe that we all perceive differently then how we perceive defines to a large degree who we are. Having said that, you can imagine that if someone has major dysfunction with vision or visual processing skills – this contributes to the inability to make eye contact or establish and maintain relationships because who you are and how you interpret the world around you is simply different. For example, if you perceive a kitten as a tiger, a pet that is perceived as cute and fun to a non-autistic child, is misperceived as dangerous to the autistic child. Vision therapy helps to alter these frightening perceptions and fosters better grounding with everyday environment. Recall the example of the automated sliding glass doors discussed earlier in this chapter.

Pat Wyman is a learning expert, teacher and founder of HowToLearn.com. She is also co-author of two books about autism. In *The Official Autism 101 Manual*, coauthored with Karen Simmons, she describes autism in the following way: "People with autism have difficulty processing and responding to information from their senses." Again, readers are encouraged to access these references for further information that will undoubtedly be helpful.

Vision is the dominant sense and 80% of a person's interpretation of the world. Because of the visual dominance in understanding and interpretation, this raises many questions about the importance of how the autistic individual processes and then responds to visual data.

Is it possible that people with autism see things differently than we do? Of course it is possible! Very few people see things identically and perception is not standardized among individuals. In fact many autistic individuals turn their head to one side or look out of the corners of their eyes. Frequently a program of vision therapy, with or without the use of ambient lenses, is very helpful. This type of noninvasive therapeutic intervention allows the patient to process, and more importantly, interpret the world around them differently. In some cases, changes are noticed immediately.

It is vital to understand that children with autism may have normal eyesight (20/20), yet benefit from one on one, office based vision therapy by a qualified vision therapy fellow.

The ability to organize visual space and gain peripheral stability is one of the goals of vision therapy for the person with autism. This aspect of vision therapy allows the patient with autism to better attend and appreciate central vision and gain more efficient eye teaming (binocular coordination) and visual information processing. Another important aspect is the ability to understand and move in space.

Most of us really don't appreciate or understand the role that vision plays in our lives. What we see defines, to a large extent, who we are. Therefore, if we change how and what we see, significant changes occur in the individual's interpretation and understanding of the world around them. This in turn, allows the autistic child to function in a different manner. Patients, with whom we have worked, usually make very good progress as reported to us from their parents.

It is important to decide which therapies might be most helpful with each individual. Remember that each child is different as are their needs. With the appropriate interventions, the autistic child can be helped. To that end, behavioral optometrists, as licensed professionals, are among the most committed doctoral trained clinicians to step up to the plate to help children with autism.

REFERENCES

www.webmd.com/brain/autism/tc/aspergers-syndrome-symptoms *(Last accessed: July 19, 2012)*

www.mayoclinic.com/health/autism *(Last accessed: July 19, 2012)*

www.aswtcc.org *(Last accessed: July 19, 2012)*

American Psychiatric Association. Pervasive developmental disorders. In: Diagnostic and Statistical Manual of Mental Disorders (4th ed.---text revision (DSM-IV-TR). Washington, DC: American Psychiatric Association 2000:69-70.)

RECOMMENDED READING

Greenspan S. Engaging Autism Using the Floortime Approach to Help Children Relate, Communicate, and Think. Cambridge, MA: Da Capo Press, 2006.

Greenspan S, Wieder S, Robin Simons R. The Child With Special Needs: Encouraging Intellectual and Emotional Growth. New York: Perseus Books, 1998.

Kaplan M. Seeing through New Eyes. London: Jessica Kingsley Publishers, 2006.

Temple G, Scariano Margaret M. Emergence: Labeled Autistic. Novato, CA: Arena Press, 1986.

Temple G Thinking In Pictures and Other Reports From My Life With Autism. New York: Vintage Books, 2006.

CHAPTER 8
THE WORKPLACE AND COMPUTER VISION SYNDROME (CVS)

Tarzan sits all day in a tiny cubicle staring into a computer screen. That picture sums up the plight of the many people who work in an environment that is not user friendly to the very nature of human vision.

As we know, in this age of technology, most people earn their living doing some kind of deskwork. Among them are many whose eyes, adapted to distant vision, will suffer to a greater or lesser degree from focusing all day at arm's length. For an increasing number of people, close work involves staring at a computer screen for part or all of the day. While technology and computerized devices have advanced the world in many ways, the back-lit screen has stressed all aspects of vision and made a bad visual situation considerably worse.

An article published in the *Los Angeles Times* (July 20, 2008) called public attention to the notion that scientifically valid studies have shown that 35 to 90% of people who spend 3 or more hours on the computer have eye disorders. In addition, those who use bifocal or progressive lenses have increased chances of developing Computer Vision Syndrome (CVS). Let's take a look at some of the facts.

The average computer user at work spends 950 hours a year in front of a computer. Another 300 hours are spent in front of their home computer for a total of about 156 eight hour workdays a year in front of a backlit screen at close range. (Source: National Science Board, Science and Engineering Indicators, 2000)

It was estimated that by the year 2005 at least 20% of the US workforce would be telecommuting from home through a computer. In addition 89 million US employees are online on a daily basis at work. (*Newsweek*, April 30, 2001)

It is estimated that 60 million Americans suffer from CVS, a condition that continues to remain unknown to consumers. According to the US Census Bureau, 175 million adults and children use computers. Of this number, 90% of youths between the ages of 9 and 17 use computers, putting them at very high risk for CVS. (www. eyes.org. Last accessed: November 2011)

CVS is an increasing concern both in the schools system as well as in the workplace, so much so that it has resulted some states developing workplace guidelines or legislation. Florida, Nebraska, Rhode Island, West Virginia, New York and Massachusetts are among some of the states that have enacted legislation requiring children to pass comprehensive vision exams before moving on in school or if they have been diagnosed with a developmental learning delay problem.

In Massachusetts, proof of a comprehensive pre-school visual exam by a licensed optometric physician or ophthalmologist is necessary before the child is admitted into the school system. As momentum for paying attention to the vast amount of hidden and overlooked vision related problems that plaque the US, federal legislation provides grants for the development of vision programs for high risk children. In New York, the New York Children's Vision Coalition provides comprehensive eye exams to New York City school students in underachieving schools. Of the 322 children who received the exams, 39% were found to need further vision care.

The state of Maine enacted legislation requiring employers to provide training in the proper use of computer screens, vision exams in the first six months of employment at a new job followed by mandatory annual vision exams (http://www.maine.gov/labor/workplace_safety/publications/VDTbooklet.pdf). Meanwhile the Department of Health in New Jersey has also enacted a voluntary program that offers recommendations concerning VDT use and eye exams. www.state.nj.us/health/eoh/peoshweb/vdtgpt1.pdf. At least 19 other states have introduced legislation concerning computer use.

Approximately 50% of computer users in the United States have some level of CVS according to Jim Sheedy, OD, PhD, head of the Vision Ergonomics Research Laboratory and Professor of Optometry at Pacific University. According to Dr. Sheedy, 60-90% of computer users experienced eye and vision disorders. The eyestrain experiences are related not only to the backlit screens from computers but also to other electronic gadgets. This increased visual concentration exacerbates convergence insufficiencies and other binocular dysfunction creating symptoms of visual stress.

A survey of optometrists conducted by Sheedy revealed that general symptoms of ocular discomfort after computer use were more intense and more frequent. These symptoms included eyestrain, headache, eye fatigue, as well as general overall fatigue. Specific vision disorders include blurred distant vision after computer use, development of myopia (nearsightedness), accommodative disorder symptoms and diplopia or double vision.

Paying attention to these health issues is most important for not only individuals but to workplace environments as well, since work efficiency decreases dramatically when employees experience CVS.

An Internet press release (http:/mytechnoguide.com/2010/09/use-right-font-to-avoid-burning-eyes-new-study-in-us) in August of 2010 revealed that in India more than 75% of the young software professionals as well as technical students face vision disorders that stem from the increasing use of laptops, mobile internet and other technology gadgets that strain the eye. While we refer to this most recent press release, there are countless articles in the media on CVS.

Symptoms related to CVS include temporary weak vision, dry, irritated eyes, light sensitivity, tiredness, soreness, dry eyes, redness, fatigue, repeated headaches, burning of the eyes, pain in and around the eyes, sensitivity to glare, difficulty focusing, contact lens difficulty, periodic blurring or near or distant vision, excessive tearing, general eye strain and/or double vision.

With all of this in the news, lets take a look at some case examples. David H is an editor. As a nearsighted person, he has worn glasses since his early teens, and now, in his 60s, his glasses are now bifocals. He has been an avid reader since childhood. Doing his work successfully depends first of all on his ability to read rapidly and comfortably for hours on end. Much of his time is spent in front of a computer screen. Until recently, reading presented no problem. He read all day at his work and then would spend the evening reading for pleasure.

In his early 60s, David noticed that his capacity for reading was diminishing. In the late afternoon his eyes would begin to feel uncomfortable. His sight would blur so that it was both difficult and painful to follow the words on the page. His right eye was particularly troublesome. It was sore and teary; it didn't seem to function properly much of the time. When he was tired, his eyes drifted apart and he was seeing a double image. He was fidgety and restless, yet forced himself to go on working. Some days he would simply give up and it got to the point where he was giving up leisure reading. Now in the evening he would put down his book after a couple of pages and wander around looking for something to do. He found his productivity falling and feared that his income would follow suit.

Our examination showed that David had divergence excess which means that his eyes turned out easily, and that he found it increasingly difficult to turn his eye inward. David was seeing with both eyes only intermittently; much of the time his weaker right eye was not even functioning. This is the beginning of amblyopia, the loss of sight in one eye because the brain, to rid itself of an unwanted double image, rejects one of the images. Untreated, this can result in severe loss of sight in the rejected eye.

After six months of therapy, David's vision was much improved. Most of his vision therapy activities were designed to give him better control over his eye movements. With other therapeutic activities his eyes worked separately, so that in order to see the whole picture he was forced to use both eyes. This was intended to induce the brain to register the messages of the weak right eye. He began to report improvement after three months and after another three said that he was now content with his vision. He said he was once more able to put in a full day at his desk without discomfort and read in the evening besides. He no longer felt his eyes drifting apart, and his sight seldom blurred. His right eye no longer bothered him. It didn't get irritated late in the day, and he didn't have the feeling that it was not seeing as well as his left eye. Our tests confirmed these reports: he was better able to manage his eye movements, and the intermittent suppression of sight in the right eye was gone. The sight in his right eye was improved. His two eyes saw equally well with the same prescription he'd had when he started vision therapy.

Much of the improvement in David's vision was due to the control his therapy gave him over the coordination of his eyes. He also practiced strategies suggested for minimizing visual stress. His desk, fortunately, is by a big window with a view that stretches off for a couple of miles. David now makes it a practice to stop every so often, lift his eyes, and gaze out the window at the most distant objects he can see. He need not interrupt his train of thought; he can think about what he's doing while he gazes at the horizon. He has learned also that he can dispel occasional blurring by shifting his focus rapidly back and forth between the words on the page and a painting on the wall. These two strategies, gazing away and shifting focus, clear his sight and allow him to go on working without discomfort.

Dentists work under conditions of potentially high visual stress. They need excellent eye-hand coordination and, above all, accurate depth perception to gauge the very small distances within which they work. Failing depth perception brought one dentist to our office for vision therapy.

Ervin N was 38 when he first noticed the signs that his depth perception was not as good as it had been. When he placed sutures after a surgery, he was having trouble finding the end of the thread. When giving an injection he would sometimes miss the mark by a few millimeters. Sometimes when he was tired he would see double. In retrospect Ervin realized that he had been avoiding the use of his left eye. He would seat himself in relation to the patient so as to rely on his right eye. "I was going very monocular," he recalled. That was the root of his problem, since binocular vision (both eyes working as a team) is what makes depth perception possible.

We found that his eyes were doubly turned. Both eyes drifted outward, while his left eye would also turn upward. He was getting a double form of double vision: double images, separated both from side to side and up and down. Keeping a single image was a constant struggle.

Ervin began a course of vision therapy that lasted six months. The therapy eliminated his lateral strabismus: his eyes no longer tended to drift outward. But vertical strabismus does not always respond to therapy and his left eye still turned upward. During his vision therapy, we compensated for the upward turn by adding a prism to the prescription in his glasses.

The therapy strengthened Ervin's left eye and thus helped him makes his two eyes work as a team. He no longer avoided use of his left eye, and his occasional double vision disappeared. Most important, he no longer experienced any visual problem in his work. Ervin once more had the excellent depth perception that his profession requires.

So far we have discussed visual problems as they apply to the individual, but in some occupations an untreated visual defect can also be a hazard to the general public. In the case of an airline pilot, the point needs no further explanation. The same applies to the much larger numbers of people who highway drive for a living or those who drive extensively for leisure, a subject addressed in Chapter 9. Dentists and surgeons whose vision is troubled are more likely to make mistakes with serious consequences for their patients. In all these examples, the problem is not necessarily with the person's sight. Visual stress leaves a person in less than the best condition to make vital decisions. Dentists and surgeons who suffer from headaches, eyestrain or general tension because of the visual environment are not going to be performing at their best when the critical moment comes, even when their eye exam checks out perfectly on the eye chart.

Far less familiar is the case of the radiologist. Radiologists are the medical doctors who read our X rays and, on the basis of what they see there, decide if there is a problem that needs medical attention. In many cases that reading of the X ray is the decisive factor in whether the patient gets timely treatment.

Studies of the readings made by radiologists have produced results that are truly alarming. (Tuddenham 1962, Yerushalmy J 1969) Three steps go into reading an X ray: taking the film, perceiving what it shows, and interpreting that evidence. The first and third steps the technology of taking the picture and the interpretation of the evidence have received considerable attention. The second step, perception, has been little studied, and yet it is there that most mistakes are made.

In 1977 radiologist, Dr. Frederick Taber, summarized the results of a series of studies. One study compared five radiologists' interpretations of the same 1,256 X-ray films. The difference in their positive diagnoses ("positive" meaning a problem that needed attention) ranged from a low of 56 to a high of 100, with the other three in between. Three months later the same five radiologists were asked to read the same X rays again. Now each radiologist disagreed with his own previous reading of the positive cases one time in five on the average.

Startled by this outcome, two other researchers staged their own experiments and got similar results. In another study, this time of chest X rays, the researcher found that eight radiologists and chest specialists missed one-quarter of the cases that another expert panel had found were "clinically urgent." In still another study, two radiologists disagreed in 30% of the cases, and each one on later reading disagreed with him 20% of the time.

All this is bound to be disturbing, if not downright terrifying, to anyone whose life may hang on a radiologist's reading of his or her X ray. One researcher, speaking to fellow radiologists, offered self-defense evidence that other forms of medical diagnosis are at least as prone to error as radiology. That may be of some comfort to radiologists, but obviously it does nothing at all for the rest of us.

Not all job related vision problems involve close work. The large category of strabismus (turned eye) and amblyopia (lazy eye) can make life difficult for people whose occupation does not center on reading or other kinds of arm's-length work.

These two problems together affect 5 to 6% of the United States population. As we noted earlier, orthoptics, the ancestor of today's vision therapy, was born in the early nineteenth century when the French ophthalmologist Emile Javal rebelled against the surgery then practiced for strabismus. But the surgical treatment persisted, and still persists today, despite the vast accumulation of evidence showing that it frequently provides dismal results. Surgery can often correct the cosmetic problem, but in the great majority of patients it does not correct the patient's visual problems. The eye that was turned may now appear to be properly aligned, but the patient still does not have adequate binocular vision: the two eyes do not work together as a team. The eyes look right but do not work right. In the large number of people who suffer from strabismus without a visibly turned eye, surgery is unlikely to be of any help at all since there being no cosmetic problem to correct, and would only weaken the muscles of the eye.

Yet all too often surgery is still practiced in such cases. An example is Gretchen S: Gretchen was in her early 40s when she began to have very serious trouble with her vision. She wore glasses for nearsightedness, but glasses could not correct her new problems. When she tried to look down, her eyes would not work together and she saw double. She had to tip her head to one side to get a single image and then her neck began to ache. She could go downstairs only by closing one eye and holding on to a railing. She could read, only by holding the paper straight out in front of her. She found herself bumping into things, and she suffered occasional falls. Driving was difficult and chancy; she had two accidents in one year.

Worst of all, Gretchen found herself unable to function in her work as a physical therapist. Her peripheral vision had become so poor she could not keep track of what was going on in a room full of her patients. She could not keep up with the necessary paperwork. Reluctantly, she gave up a career she loved and had the experience and took up less visually demanding work as a massage therapist.

In her desperate search for help Gretchen made the rounds of eye doctors. An ophthalmologist recommended surgery, and she was operated on as he had recommended. The surgery helped somewhat, she said, but the basic problems remained unchanged. She still could not look down more than 20° to 30° without seeing double. "It was not what I'd hoped for," she recalled. Again she consulted a series of eye specialists. Again they had nothing to recommend but more surgery. Again she was operated on one month later. She felt that the second surgery changed nothing at all, and she felt that all of her problems were equally as bad as before. Once more she made the rounds to a string of doctors. Another surgeon recommended yet another surgery with a prognosis of a "50-50" chance of success. But Gretchen rebelled at that prospect. She kept on asking and eventually a psychologist working in vocational rehabilitation suggested she try vision therapy, and she came to our office for help. The hardest part was telling her that with the damage done to her eye muscles by the two surgeries affected her chances of a successful outcome and she was told that no promises could be made.

"You got the biggest piece," said the girl. Nobody answered. Nobody looked at the little fairy "Both of you got more than I did," The children were looking Said the smallest child. "I want more!" at their plates. The three children howled. The "You got the piece of turkey I wanted. mother scolded. The father beat said the boy. on the table with a spoon. What a noise! "You got the biggest piece," said the "This cannot be Thanksgiving," girl. said the fairy. "This is not fun. "Both of you got more than I did," I do not like it.

DOUBLE VISION

Simulation of person seeing double while reading.

Vertical imbalance like Gretchen's is quite hard to treat. Such an imbalance combined with the negative effects of surgery made her potentially one of our most difficult cases. She decided to try anyway, and we started a course of vision therapy.

After six months Gretchen's vision was considerably improved. Her eyes worked together better, and she could look down as much as 40° without seeing double. She could read without holding the paper as high as she did before, and she could tolerate more paperwork. Her peripheral vision, still limited, was considerably improved. Driving was less difficult, but she still had to be extra careful while behind the wheel. She felt more confident and was not so unhappy with her vision. "I have much more confidence when I use my eyes," she said. "Life is not nearly as stressful as it was." She estimated that her vision had come about one-half of the way back to what it had been before her troubles began.

Gretchen felt bitter by the 'bum steer' in consenting to surgery, not once, but twice, and she felt angry with the surgeons who performed them. She recalls that she asked the surgeons time and again if there were any exercises she could do that might help her vision, a natural question for a physical therapist to ask. Always the answer was no. "Why didn't they tell me about vision therapy?" she asks.

A special category among people with job-related visual problems includes those who take up a visually demanding career after years spent in another kind of life. Typically these are women who have spent most of their 20s and 30s raising a family and working full time, at home. Demanding as that life surely is it does not take a lot of intense close visual work. If such a person returns to work, or often school followed by work, she may find that her vision is not up to the sudden new demand for a lot of arm's length visual concentration. An example is Julie O.

Julie had raised three children when she decided to go back to work. The career in family therapy that she wanted to pursue meant she would have to earn a master's degree, and then enter a doctoral program that would require a great deal more reading than she had had to do in college. Once she was a full time student again, after many years away from the books, she found she was having trouble with the quantity of graduate school reading. Her attention span was limited. It was hard to focus in the mornings and because she had to put so much energy into focusing her eyes, she did not have enough energy left to focus in the intellectual sense. She worried about the years of even heavier reading that lay ahead. Could she keep up with her much younger fellow students?

We found that Julie had a mild form of divergent strabismus: one eye drifted out from time to time. Julie committed to 20 hours of vision therapy over the summer, before she entered her doctoral program.

Julie found that she could function better as a student after her therapy. Her eyes no longer bothered her when she was studying. The problem of focusing in the mornings vanished. "Because I no longer had to think about my eyes, I had much more energy to think about the subject," she said. She could read for longer periods at a stretch, with much greater comfort.

Like David H, she took to heart our advice on ways to limit visual stress when she was studying. She would take regular breaks during which she would gaze out her window at the buildings across the street. She discovered that these breaks did not hinder but actually helped her learning. Shifting the focus of her attention gave her a wider perspective on her work. By looking up from the 'single tree' on the page before her, she was able, while gazing away, to see the 'forest' of the subject that was the real focus of her attention. In time Julie got her doctoral degree and went into practice as a family therapist.

Computer screens magnify and multiplies the visual problems of deskwork. As we have an ever increasing demand for computerized tasks in everyday life, the number of people suffering from vision problems grows and they complain at a greater rate than their counterparts who are working only with paper related tasks.

Reading from a computer screen, iPod or Kindle is not just another form of reading since electronic and printed images differ in quality than those that are printed on a hardcopy. A given sentence is harder to read on a backlit screen than on the printed page. Whereas the printed copy is clear and still, the backlit image is comparatively blurred and is constantly moving and flickering. Dr. Lawrence Stark, a neurologist member of a National Academy of Science committee on the impact of video display, said: "VDTs require much more of the visual system than any other office related visual tasks . . . . VDT characters are not as readable as printed material." The VDT has also made visual work more concentrated by changing the way many jobs are performed. The more steps of the job that can be performed on the VDT, the less respite the operator gets from staring at the terminal. The data entry clerk is an example. Before computers, he would take orders by telephone, and then write them up by hand or typewriter on an order form. The person assisting you often had to carry papers to other desks or offices. Thus he or she had frequent cause to interrupt close visual work. Not with the computer screen or backlit screen. That same clerk now wears a phone headset and enters all information directly into the terminal. This type of work provides few if any visual breaks.

In our practice we are seeing a fast growing number of patients who spend their working days in front of a backlit screen. Their complaints fall into patterns. Their sight blurs, they see double, they have trouble changing focus when they look away from the screen. Their eyes burn and ache. They feel eyestrain and visual fatigue. They have frequent headaches, especially of the forehead.

Certainly, as we have seen, these same complaints have often been voiced by those who work with printed hard copy materials, but not to quite the degree as we see with intense long hours spent in front of a backlit screen. Some patients have told us they had no trouble with deskwork until they started working with backlit screens. Several studies have shown a much higher rate of visual complaints among backlit screen users than among other types of deskwork. One study compared the rate of complaint in five categories:

WORKPLACE VISUAL COMPLAINTS

COMPLAINT	Percent VDT workers	Percent non-VDT clerical workers
Change in color perception	40	9
Irritated eyes	74	47
Burning eyes	80	44
Blurred vision	71	35
Eyestrain	91	60

Patients tell us their visual problems have a direct and harmful effect on their work and on their general health. They cannot work as fast or as well or get as much done in a day. They make more errors in transcribing words and numbers, more reversals, omissions, substitutions. Visual fatigue leads to physical fatigue and visual stress leads to overall stress making one more susceptible to illness: virus, colds, allergies.

And employers take note that our patients lose more days out sick. Many corporate managers have instituted wellness programs for their employees in the belief that better employee health means a healthier balance sheet. We believe that employers would be wise to include vision in their wellness programs. Such a program would include regular examinations and not merely the standard Snellen chart, but also include a full range of visual skills and support the need for vision therapy where

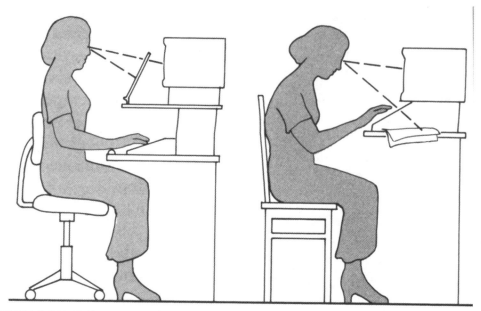

VIDEO DISPLAY TERMINAL WORKSTATIONS

Note the contrasts between the well-designed station, left, and one that is poorly designed. At left, the chair provides support for the back and its height is adjustable so that the operator can maintain good posture and can keep her feet flat on the floor. Both the video screen and the document to the right of the screen are at about a forearm's length from the eyes and about 20-30 degrees below eye level. The height of the adjustable table is set so that the operator's forearms and wrists are approximately horizontal while using the keyboard, and so her legs clear the underside of the table.

indicated. The figures on the effects of close work on employees persuade us that such a program would easily pay for itself in improved productivity and reduced absenteeism.

Again, statistics confirm what we observe among our patients. An Air Force study of office automation found a high degree of complaints such as head and backaches, even arm and leg pains, along with directly visual complaints such as eyestrain. A survey of 1,000 members of the Newspaper Guild found that "more VDT users than non-users said they had been absent from work three or more times in the preceding two years." An eye clinic specializing in VDT operators the Video Display Terminal Eye Clinic in Berkeley, California has found that an unusually large number of its patients have trouble focusing their eyes.

Much of the human discomfort and suffering these statistics represent is unnecessary. There are ways to reduce the visual and physical impact of the VDT. These fall into two categories: improving the conditions in which VDT operators work, and helping the operators improve their visual skills so they can better handle the visual burden of technology.

Most computer operators work in circumstances that fall far short of the ideal. Proper conditions begin with the right arrangement of the operator in relation to the machine. The chair supports the back and is adjustable so the operator can keep both feet flat on the floor. The seat pad is set so that the person's legs are 1-2" from the chair with back against the backrest. The forearms and wrists are approximately horizontal while using the keyboard. The display screen is above the keyboard, about arm's length (18-20") from the operator's eyes, and 20°-30° below his direct line of sight. (Why below rather than straight ahead? As in so many aspects of vision, the answer goes back to our remote ancestors. When they were working with their hands, whether cracking nuts or tearing meat from the carcass, they too were looking down rather than straight ahead.)

Glare and reflection must be minimized. Ideally, the display screen should have a neutral matte finish. A filter can also be put over the screen. Operators should avoid wearing light colored clothes, which, combined with the light given off by the screen, cause both glare and reflection.

Resolution, the visual quality of the display on the screen, is determined by the density of the phosphorescent dots, called pixels, which when electronically excited form the images we see. (The same is true of a television screen.) The higher the resolution that is, the greater the concentration of pixels, the better it is for the eyes. "Swim" (the slight waving motion of the image) and on-off flickering are subtly harmful to the eyes. Getting a machine of good quality can minimize both and then making sure it is well maintained.

Thinking about the right colors on the screen has changed since the early days of computers. The makers of the first screens used the familiar black and white. This provided good contrast, as it does on paper, but on computer screens, the combination of black and white is fatiguing to the eyes.

Lighting requirements change when work moves from paper to the backlit screens because the operator needs only half the lighting needed by someone who would be working with paper. What used to be the right amount of illumination in the room is likely now to be too much. Because today's screen is higher in relation to our eyes than yesterday's paper, overhead glare will be more bothersome. Diffuse, indirect lighting is preferable. Fluorescent lights provide this, but, for reasons of eye health having nothing to do with backlit screens, they should be the full-spectrum kind. Natural light from a window is valuable as a source of visual relief, but can cause glare if their light falls directly on the screen.

People who work on backlit screens must have ample and frequent opportunity to take breaks from the near-point visual concentration of their work. Ideally, they should have five to ten minutes every hour away from the machine. That time away from the terminal should not be spent in any other kind of close visual activity such as reading a newspaper or even glancing through a magazine.

The purpose of a break is to give workers a chance to cast their eyes off into the distance, so there must be an opportunity for that distant view. Even a brief glance far away from the terminal helps reduce the strain on the eyes. That is why windows are valuable.

That essential distant view is denied by those employers who, in order to save space, put their staff in tiny cubicles where their visual space is as little as 4'. The person working in that cubicle has no relief from the stress of his or her close work on the terminal. The result is not one of the best. Whatever else is being produced in those cubicles, one product is certain: nearsightedness. The work cubicle is where we are likely to find the person whose myopia leveled off in their early twenties and now in their thirties it is suddenly getting worse again. Here, too, we will find the person who is becoming nearsighted for the first time.

Employers may save money on the rent by herding employees into those visual sweatshops, but they will pay a high price in lower productivity on the job and more days out sick. It is likely, in our view, that the employer would be better off paying more rent in order to get more production from healthier, happier workers. For the employees themselves, there is no doubt they would be better off, much better off, out of the cubicles.

Only so much can be done to improve the work environment. A comparison of the rates of vision problems under best and worst conditions suggests that the best environment will reduce complaints by up to 39%. Better resolution on the screen, reduces complaints at a rate of around 11%. Most backlit screen problems are due to the visual limitations of the operators themselves and must be resolved with glasses or vision therapy or a combination of the two.

People who already wear glasses will most likely need a new prescription as they continue to work with backlit screens. The usual prescription, intended to provide 20/20 eyesight on the chart, is often poorly adapted to use in front of backlit screens. In fact, in many cases, a separate prescription just for computer use would be found helpful. Computer glasses should be designed for use at the distance from the eyes to the computer. It would also be helpful if the worker measured that distance before seeing the eye doctor since this is very important information for the examining doctor. If the doctor says this information is not necessary, perhaps you may have the wrong doctor.

This is particularly true of the middle-aged person who wears bifocals. Because the display screen is both higher and farther away, a person of this age cannot read as they normally would with bifocals. In this situation it is necessary to tilt the head back to look at the screen through the lower lenses. Pretty soon the neck is aching. This situation and that of others wearing glasses can be remedied with special glasses for the backlit screen user. In recent years lenses have been developed, often with a single or variable focus, which can be tailored to the specific needs of the job. Anyone who already wears glasses and uses computers extensively is well advised to ask an eye doctor for work glasses and to give the doctor the most precise description possible of the visual requirements of their job, especially the exact distance between the eyes and the screen.

Once more, research confirms the observations we have made in our practice. Two optometrists at the State College of Optometry in New York, Dr. Barry J. Barresi and Dr. Jesse Rosenthal, reported on 775 computer workers who were given special eye tests by a panel of optometrists. Seventy five percent were given glasses tailored to their jobs. Among those who answered a follow-up questionnaire, 94% reported greater comfort and 82% said the quality and efficiency of their work had improved. The researchers observed that people over 40 years of age seemed to benefit the most. It should also be noted that many of the over 40 patients also wore corrective glasses.

Visually, a computer screen is far more demanding than other kinds of deskwork. It requires high performance in eye movements, in binocular vision, and in the ability to focus for long stretches and then change focus without blurring. If a person's skills in these areas are mediocre, they will experience discomfort working for any length of time in front of the screen. If their skills are poor, the handicap will be severe. Vision therapy will bring this person's skills up to the point where, given good working conditions, they can do a full day's work without discomfort. Vision therapy can also enhance skills that are already good. For the person whose skills are good enough for most daily uses, therapy can raise the level of those skills so that work completed on backlit screens with greater ease and efficiency.

Lets look at a case example: Jean A is a software developer in her late 20s. Her work is very demanding on her vision. She spends 80% of her working day looking at the screen, and the rest of her day is devoted to close deskwork.

Her eye doctor referred her to us. She told us that her eyes were tiring; she was seeing double, she was missing whole paragraphs when she read and she was suffering from frequent headaches. She also mentioned that she had been operated on at age 13 for an eye that turned out.

We found that the surgery Jean had gone through overcorrected her eye so that instead of turning out it now turned in. Her brain was intermittently suppressing the messages from that eye and when it did accept those messages, Jean was seeing double. We suggested a course of therapy and prescribed work glasses that include a prism to help hold her eye in line and are coated to screen out ultraviolet radiation.

After a year of therapy, plus eight weeks of reinforcement two years later, Jean finds that her vision is much improved. Her turned eye is straight, and she no longer sees double or suppresses one eye. She has no trouble with close work. She no longer has headaches or misses paragraphs. Most importantly, she can do a day's work in front of a backlit screen without the trouble she used to have. She also made it a habit to take regular breaks, every 45 minutes or so, to relieve the visual concentration of her work. After vision therapy Jean was rewarded with enough visual energy after a full day of intense work and still be able to enjoy reading at home in the evening.

Vincent L is another case example. Vincent is an electronics technician. He repairs computer related equipment of various sorts. Some of his tasks involve intricate work with tiny wires calling for good eye-hand coordination. Most of his day is spent either staring into a computer screen or reading small type in thick manuals.

When he was 30, Vincent began to feel very uncomfortable in his work. Reading the manuals was especially frustrating. He could not get through the instructions at one sitting. He would read a page, then feel he had to stop and get up. He was beginning to guess at the instructions or rely on what he had heard. He did whatever he needed in order to avoid reading the manual. He got a headache at the prospect of paper work. He had trouble judging where things were in space. Reading had always made him uncomfortable. Never a good reader or speller, he had gotten through high school by listening carefully. Later his poor reading had caused him to drop out of one school after another. Now he was unpleasantly aware of a disparity between what he produced and the work of others. He wasn't working up to his ability and he knew it. He tried glasses, but this, he said, was "worse than nothing." Then he was referred to us.

When we examined Vincent we found he suffered from convergence insufficiency: he found it difficult to align his eyes on a close target and hold them there. His visual skills were those of a fourth grader. We gave him a reading comprehension test, in which, in his own words, he "did pretty horrible." We proposed therapy to improve his visual skills. We also prescribed glasses that corrected his farsightedness and astigmatism without causing discomfort.

Vincent's therapy lasted nine months and was a complete success. His eyes now work together without difficulty. His life is greatly improved, both at work and at home. He no longer has trouble reading long reports, and he suffers no headaches or frustration in front of a computer screen. His work is much better. In fact, he has been promoted twice. His reading comprehension tests far higher than it did when he started with us: he has gone from fourth grade to college level in less than a year. He reads 325 words a minute where he used to read no more than 110. Still a poor speller, he now is willing to look a word up and get it right. He is even, for the first time in his life, reading for pleasure. He reads spy stories passed on to him by his wife.

One subtle visual skill deserves separate mention. This is the balance between central and peripheral vision, between what we see where we focus our eyes and what we are aware of in the larger surrounding area. If this relationship is properly balanced, the person working with computers or doing any other close work will be able to center their primary attention on work while maintaining a good sense of where he or she is in the environment. This allows one to be aware of what is going on around him or herself and not be distracted by surroundings. This, too, we owe to our ancestors, whose peripheral vision warned of impending danger while they focused on the immediate tasks of cracking nuts or tearing meat. If a person's attention is too peripheral they will be easily distracted by movements or surrounding sounds. If, on the other hand, they are over balanced toward the center, they will be able to concentrate but also easily fatigued.

Therapeutic exercises improve the visual balance between central and peripheral awareness. A better balance in our perception has an analogy in our mental performance. At the center our mind is focused on the most immediate part of the task, while on the periphery of the mind we are aware of the larger aspects of our work. At the center, our attention is on the present what we are doing right now. On the periphery, we are aware of past and future, in other words, what we have just done and what we are going to do next. Here, too, a better balance between the two will improve human performance, not just with backlit screens, but also in many aspects of life.

The problems associated with computerized technology will hardly diminish let alone go away. In a world ever more dependent on technology and micro management of the world, vision problem identification is ever more important. Now is the time to embrace vision therapy as a means of correcting, managing, and preventing unnecessary loss of human potential and comfort. Vision therapy can in fact, enable humans and technology to mesh in ways that will be more promising than having individual persons needlessly struggle and problem solve, unsuccessfully on their own. We have to learn to live with technology and vision therapy can be a major force in achieving human potential in our age of technology.

With the improved performance after vision therapy, it is not uncommon for the individual to be promoted and given greater responsibility, thus, often an increase in salary follows.

BIBLIOGRAPHY

Tuddenham WJ, 1962 Visual search, image organization, and reader error in roentgen diagnosis: studies of the psycho-physiology of roentgen image. Radiology 78:694-704; doi:10.1148/78.5.694.

Yerushalmy J, 1969. The statistical assessment of the variability in observer perception and description of roentgenographic pulmonary shadows. Radiol Clin North Am;7:381-92.

Sheedy JE, Shaw-McMinn PG, 2003. Diagnosing and Treating Computer-Related Vision Problems. Boston: Butterworth Book Publishers.

Sheedy JE, 1992. Vision problems at video display terminals: A survey of optometrists. J Am Optom Assoc;63:687-92.

Chapter 9
Driving and Household Accidents

Driving is one modern activity for which our ancestors were in many ways visually well prepared. In most of this book we have been discussing visual skills needed for close work, skills for which the eyes we inherited from our ancestors are poorly adapted. Driving, by contrast, calls on the same skills that our ancestors needed in order to find their food and at the same time escape becoming a meal for a hungry predator.

Peter B was one of our most unusual and challenging cases. Most patients come to us with more or less severe visual problems. Not Peter. His vision was excellent, his visual skills far above average. The challenge he posed was to make his excellent skills even better.

Peter, who is in his 30s, is a serious amateur race car driver. Almost any weekend from spring through fall finds him out on one track or another racing against his peers. He has never had serious problems with his eyes. In graduate school, when he was reading six to eight hours a day, he'd notice his sight blurring occasionally. He got reading glasses, but hasn't worn them since graduation because his profession does not require concentrated close work. On the racetrack, however, Peter is an intense competitor. He'd heard of vision therapy and wondered if it could improve his vision and thereby his racing. "It wasn't enough for my vision to work right," he said later. "I wanted it to work just right. I wanted the last one percent."

We examined Peter and found that, excellent as his skills were, some aspects of his vision were less than perfect. The Brock String tests spatial judgment: the patient reaches out to touch a point on a string that the therapist holds perpendicular to his eyes. Peter would reach slightly beyond the actual location of the point. He was seeing things like other race cars somewhat further away than they really were, so he was reacting a split second late. When his eyes tired, as they would late in a long race, he would have trouble refocusing and would lose a little of his intense concentration. We told him we could try to help him to gain that last 1% of his vision. Peter entered a course of therapy in which we concentrated on those few skills that could be improved. He came to us two hours a week for four months. Of his therapy, he recalled particularly an exercise in which he drew lines with each hand simultaneously while seeing the lines he was reproducing separately with each of his eyes.

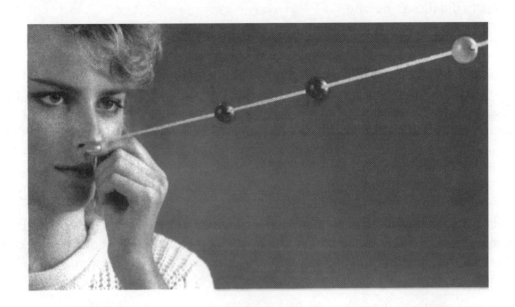

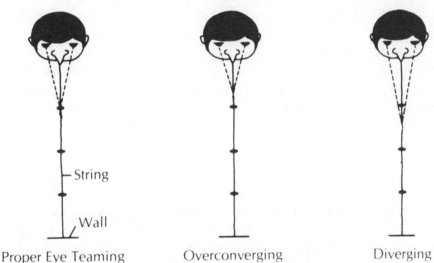

String

Wall

Proper Eye Teaming   Overconverging   Diverging

PROPER EYE TEAMING OVERCONVERGING DIVERGING

WHERE THE EYES REALLY FOCUS Testing with the "Brock String" reveals whether the eyes actually converge on the intended target. The patient holds the string as shown in the photo and is asked to focus on the bead closest to her. The string will appear to her as two converging lines. As seen in the diagram, the lines may appear to meet in front of the bead if the patient's eyes are over-converging. She will see things as being somewhat closer than they really are, and will respond according to that perception. If the lines seem to meet beyond the bead, the eyes are diverging and the patient will see things as farther away than they are. If the patient is asked to reach out and touch the bead, she will touch the string in front of the bead if her eyes overconverge, beyond it if they diverge. The judgment of distance tested by the Brock String is important in driving and in many sports.

Photo courtesy of Bernell Corporation, South Bend, Indiana

"I knew that the closer the lines came together the closer I was to seeing what's actually out there," he said.

Peter reported a noticeable improvement in his visual perception after his therapy. For him, what mattered about his therapy was what happened out on the track, and that was where he saw the difference. In his first race after therapy, he sensed an obvious improvement in his ability to concentrate visually: "I didn't have the feeling of losing concentration midway in the race." Three weeks later, racing on an unusually fast track, Peter had "a distinct impression that things were slowing down, that I had more time to react. Not much, but in a race it doesn't take much to make the difference." This is a familiar phenomenon. Many an athlete has told us after vision therapy that things, a ball he is trying to hit, for example, seem to be moving slower. Of course the ball, or in Peter's case another car is not moving with any less speed but his visual system is moving faster. It is processing information and presenting it to the brain more rapidly, and this gives the athlete an extra moment to respond. As any athlete will say a moment, even a split second, may be all it takes.

The next weekend Peter thought he was driving very well in the first day's race. The next day he spent the first 14 laps "chasing somebody." He experienced no loss of concentration. "I was giving it one hundred percent all the way," he recalled. "I sensed the moment when he was losing his visual concentration, and I caught him on the next to last lap!" He explained to us that in that moment he had hurdled a psychological barrier in racing. "Usually if you try to pass a car for several laps and fail, something inside says you can't do it; you slow down and then you'll never catch him," he said. "This time that didn't happen to me."

For his kind of driving Peter obviously needs visual skills well beyond those required by most of us as we plod along the highway. Yet even everyday driving demands a high degree of visual skill, especially in those moments of emergency that any driver must sooner or later meet. The frightening reality is that a large proportion of people licensed to drive lack those skills. The evidence is in the great number of accidents after which the driver will say something like: "I didn't see that car coming" or "I looked but I didn't see it."

Driving requires much more than good sight. What matters, after all, is not just what the driver sees but what he does with what he sees and when he does it. Thus, in addition to visual skills, he needs good visual perception to interpret what his eyes see, the ability to react in time, and good eye-hand and eye-foot coordination to carry out effectively what he's decided to do.

Unfortunately, the state authority that issues driver's licenses tests few of these skills. For those few skills that are tested, the standards are usually too low even for ordinary drivers, and, in our opinion, far too low for those like bus and truck drivers who carry extra responsibilities.

Visual acuity at distance is the only skill that is universally tested (the familiar Snellen wall chart). The usual requirement for an ordinary license is 20/40 with glasses (sometimes this applies only to one eye). Some states set a higher minimum for bus or truck licenses.

Acuity of 20/40 is truly a minimal requirement, adequate for ordinary driving by daylight. At least two studies have shown that drivers with relatively poor acuity have a greater rate of accidents. At night the difference becomes much greater. According to one authority, optometrist Merrill J. Allen (1996), author of the landmark study *Vision and Highway Safety*, that driver with 20/20 by daylight may after dark have effective sight of only 20/40; far too poor for safety.

The usual test is for static acuity, how well we see when either we, or the object we look at is, in motion. But obviously, in driving, both the driver and other cars are in motion. As we say in more detail in Chapter 11, dynamic acuity does not follow from static acuity. Unfortunately, only a handful of states test for this important skill.

Visual acuity is just the beginning of a driver's visual needs. It measures only our ability to see what we are looking at. Usually that is what is in front of us. But most highway emergencies come at us from where we are not looking. That is what makes them emergencies. Avoiding the possible accident calls on our peripheral vision, the ability to sense an unusual motion off to the side, out of the corner of the eye, just as our ancestors sensed that saber-toothed tiger creeping up on them. Peripheral vision gives us a warning to turn our eyes and identify a possible danger.

A person with normal peripheral vision has a visual field of about 180°, which means he is able to detect movement at a right angle on either side while he is focusing straight ahead. (You can test your own peripheral vision by holding your

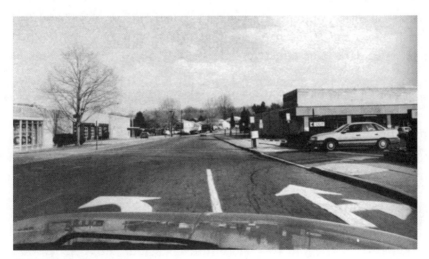

Full field standing still

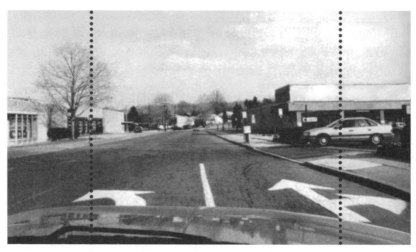

20 miles per hour

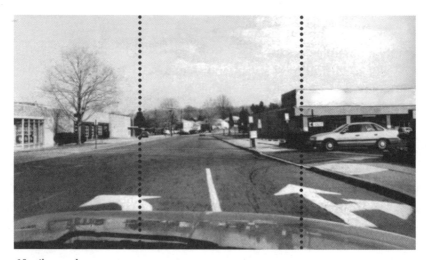

60 miles per hour

HOW SPEED DIMINISHES VISION

Peripheral vision, which extends almost to 180° when the person is motionless, decreases dramatically with increasing speed. At 20 miles an hour, a driver's peripheral vision is only 104°, and at 60, he can see only 42°–less than one-fourth his peripheral vision at rest. Note that the car at right has disappeared completely from the driver's awareness when he is going 60. He will get no warning of the car's presence until it is almost directly in front of him.

arms out to each side and wiggling your hands while looking straight ahead at a fixed target. See how far back you can move your hands before they vanish from sight.) A visual field of less than 180° is abnormal, and less than 140° is hazardous. A crucial fact here is that effective peripheral vision decreases with speed because stationary objects go by too fast to register on our eyes. Thus a visual field of 180° when standing still shrinks to 104° at 20 miles per hour and to 42° at 60 miles per hour. The driver going 60 has lost three-quarters of his peripheral vision.

Again, peripheral vision bears no relation to visual acuity. Yet few states test for it, and those few require only 140° even for bus or truck licenses.

Depth perception is another essential skill that is seldom tested. This is how we judge the distance between ourselves and another car, and act accordingly. Ideally, we judge distance with the help of binocular vision: the two eyes seeing the same object at slightly different angles give us an immediate sense of three-dimensional space. People who lack binocular vision must judge distance by using clues from other sources, for example, the space visible between two moving cars. Experience can make up for much that would otherwise come from binocularity, though probably with a loss in reaction time. The most obvious instance of a lack of binocularity is a one-eyed person, but many others also fall into this category. People with poor muscular control of their eyes find it hard to hold binocular vision. When they are tired, they may see double. When driving they can usually manage in daylight, though at some cost in fatigue and discomfort. At night, however, their vision may become unmanageable, especially under the added influence of alcohol, drugs (including medication), or exhaust fumes.

People with a turned eye (strabismus) or lazy eye (amblyopia) may have sight in both eyes but lack effective binocular vision. In *Vision and Highway Safety*, Merrill Allen identifies the person operated on for strabismus as a particular highway risk because he is likely to be less well adapted to his handicap than he was before the surgery. "Unfortunately the more hazardous surgically treated group will not be obvious to the motor vehicle examiner, while the probably safe, untreated squinter will be easy to detect," he writes. Allen believes that this surgically treated driver "should be restricted to daytime low-stress situations," whereas a turned eye "cured by non-surgical means can be considered normal."

Farsightedness is never tested, but in Allen's opinion it can be dangerous. In *Vision and Highway Safety,* he wrote: "I believe that a large proportion of one car accidents late at night result from misjudgments by young drivers who have 0.75 diopter or more of uncorrected hyperopia which is a moderate degree of farsightedness. This driver becomes confused or frightened and runs off the road when fatigued. Upon loss of the bright lights of other cars, as happens late at night, they may lose control of fusion. Fusion is the ability to keep both eyes aimed at a single object. Young drivers typically have 20/20 vision or vision better in the daytime."

Color perception is another important visual skill that is not tested routinely. Only seven states currently do so and a substantial number of people (8% of men, 0.5% of women) are deficient in their ability to distinguish color. Color deficient people have a higher rate of error while driving because the extra effort they must make to distinguish color tends to distract their attention from other aspects of driving. If their deficiency is in red and green, they will take twice as long to react to a traffic signal. Other visually related skills that are not tested are adaptability to darkness and resistance to glare (both of which diminish with age).

Visual reaction time is perhaps the most dangerous among the many omissions in our present testing of would be drivers. How quickly we are able to react is what determines how well we use all our other visual skills. Time is always short in a highway emergency, and it is no use seeing the emergency if we cannot react fast enough to avoid the accident. People vary greatly in their reaction time and this is independent of other visual skills.

Knowing that a person has excellent acuity tells us nothing about the person's ability to react to what they see. What makes this omission most unfortunate is that reaction time is easily tested and easily improved. With a little training, most people can reduce their reaction time enough to make the difference between life and death.

In order to drive safely, a complex mix of visual skills is needed. State drivers' licensing authorities would be wise to require complete vision tests in order to reduce and prevent highway accidents. We believe that states should appoint commissions that include vision experts to set higher standards not only for licensing but for driver education as well. Student drivers in particular should be tested for all the visual skills, including reaction time and peripheral vision. No student should be licensed who lacks the necessary skills, but every student ought to have access to acquiring those skills and have access to vision exams that would preempt a driving hazard.

All candidate drivers should be given that same opportunity, of course, but it is particularly easy to achieve in a school setting. We believe that making sure that all who drive have the visual skills the job requires and this would save at least as many lives as reducing speed limits from 70 to 55 miles per hour since the driver with poor skills is at least as dangerous at 55 mph as the driver with good skills would be at 70 mph.

We are aware that setting the safest standards is politically difficult. Most Americans, and particularly those who are young and male, consider a license to drive as part of their birthright. Practically speaking we live in a society for which the automobile is an essential part of daily life. For many of us it is the only way we can get to work and to the store. Driving is a privilege that must be balanced against broader social goods, namely, safety.

Still, much could be done within those limits. Minimum standards should certainly be set higher than they are today. An essential first step would be to test the full range of visual skills of all applicants for any sort of driver's license. This need not be difficult. A layman using a simple kit could test the essential skills in less than four minutes. The results of that test would form part of the driver's record and might indeed be attached to the license. Drivers' vision should be retested at regular interval and with greater frequency as they we age. All aspects of vision should be tested again after any car accident since vision may be a factor. Insurance companies might be persuaded to set different rates for different levels of skill as they do today for different age groups.

People who only meet minimum standards of vision and those who are considered visually deficient should be restricted to daytime driving. There might well be a separate test for night driving. As we have seen, visual deficiencies that are acceptable in daylight become intolerably dangerous after dark. To allow such people to drive by night is unfair not only to others, but also to themselves as well. Restricting them to daytime is a sensible compromise between the interests of safety and the rights of the individual.

The case with those who drive trucks, buses, and taxis is different. Buses and taxis carry passengers in addition to their drivers, and buses and trucks by their very size are dangerous. Truck, bus, and taxi drivers spend more time on the road, thus putting the rest of the drivers at an increased risk. The privilege to drive does not apply here any more than it does to the would-be airline pilot who cannot pass the eye exam. In the interest of the majority, applicants for these licenses should be held to high standards for the full range of visual skills. That means much higher standards than are applied today.

No doubt it will be a long time before such reforms are put into practice. In the meantime there is a lot that each the driver can do. We can begin with the awareness that we share the road with other drivers whose visual skills are deficient and that we may ourselves be among those whose vision needs therapeutic intervention. If a driver has any reason to suspect that their vision is compromised to the point where they may be more accident prone, they ought to seek professional help. It is not acceptable to say, "I didn't see that car coming." If a driver feels that they visually miss things on the road, then this should be a white flag and an excellent reason to find an eye doctor who can check the full range of their vision. If a driver finds their vision wanting for more, he should consider restricting himself to low stress daytime driving, or even take himself off the road entirely. As the old saying goes, the life he saves may be his own.

Many visual skills can be improved by conscientious practice while driving. Peter B, in an interview after his vision therapy, suggested a variety of ways in which the average driver can practice his skills and thereby prepare himself better to cope with emergency.

Avoid staring. Drivers who keep their eyes on the car in front, as if they were staring at a television screen, lose a large part of their visual field. Keep the eyes in motion. Practice rapid changes in the distance of focus—for example, switching focus from the car in front to the road far ahead and to the rearview mirror. The faster the better. The more the eyes are in motion, the better is the driver's awareness of where his vehicle is in relation to others. The less he stares, the better his peripheral vision.

Practice using the rearview mirrors, bearing in mind that distance and size are distorted in the mirrors. Try while looking at the road ahead to watch the mirrors with the "soft focus" of peripheral vision.

A driver, when driving or judging the distance and speed of cars, for example is actually practicing how to reduce reaction time; and that moment which he learns to save by practice may prove to be a lifesaver in an emergency.

To use the mirrors most effectively the driver must keep a constant position in the seat so that the each mirror can be viewed without having to look around for it. If the driver is slouched to one side, it is easy to miss the mirror on first glance. This, Peter B believes, is the primary purpose of the seat belt. Seat belts keep the driver positioned at right angles to the wheel so that the driver knows, without looking, where to find the mirrors.

Getting around the house may not seem to call for the visual skills involved in driving or the close visual work of an accountant or a dentist. But the person managing a household must carry out a wide variety of tasks that call for a variety of visual skills, and the lack of those skills spells trouble. Each year many thousands of people are injured in household accidents. Most of those accidents have a visual aspect that, if corrected, would have prevented them from happening. We tend to blame accidents on "clumsiness" and shrug them off as inevitable: that's the way the person is. But clumsiness in most cases simply means poor eye-hand coordination, and that can be improved with vision therapy.

A person with a severe visual problem can find the daily routines of life intolerably difficult. Such was the situation of Libby K. Libby's vision was in bad shape when she came to our office for professional help. Her vision was so bad, that we wondered how she could get around at all. From what she told us about her life it was clear that just getting around was indeed very hard for her.

Libby had had trouble with her vision as a child. She was always jittery when she had to study. She jumped around the page while she was reading. An eye doctor gave her a magnifying lens, which helped a little. Because she was unusually intelligent, she was able to get through high school despite her poor reading, though she recalls she was always nervous during tests. At college she majored in music and dance. She loved to dance, but she also chose it to minimize the reading she would have to do.

Later she was married and had two children. She ran a dance program for young children. With no close work to do, she was more or less free of visual problems for many years. However, when she reached her mid-40s, Libby's vision suddenly became much worse. Her ability to compensate for visual defects began to deteriorate rapidly. The activities of daily life that she had taken for granted became nearly impossible. "I was virtually nonfunctional," she recalled. "I was seeing double. My eyes were jumping all around." She could hardly read at all, and then only by using a ruler to follow the lines.

Libby had enjoyed knitting; now she could no longer knit or thread a needle. She bumped her head into kitchen cabinets. Driving became hazardous. When she backed her car out she would suddenly lose her sight and run off the driveway. She couldn't stand to look at a patterned rug. Libby even had to give up the dancing that she loved so much. Her balance was so bad she could not turn or jump without falling down. She was afraid to take off her glasses without closing her eyes because that meant seeing double. "I was always complaining," she said. "So many little things went wrong." She was nervous, high-strung and unhappy.

After a thorough visual examination, we found that Libby suffered from strabismus. Her right eye tended to turn in, and there was also a vertical imbalance between the two eyes. We started her on an intensive course of vision therapy: twice a week for five months. After her therapy Libby's vision was much improved. Her eye no longer appeared to turn. Her life was also much improved and she began to read again. "It's still not easy," she said. "But I can read short articles in the paper." She no longer bumps her head into kitchen cabinets. She can drive without running off the driveway or hitting the curb. Most important, she has started dancing again. When she is tired her vision may falter and she has to stop and rest her eyes. Overall she feels her life is far better off than it had been and her daily routine is no longer traumatic. "My husband notices the change in me," she said. "I'm much more relaxed these days. I can dance again."

REFERENCE

Allen MJ, Abrams BS, Ginsburg AP, Weintraub L. 1996. Forensic Aspects of Vision and Highway Safety. Tucson, AZ: Lawyers & Judges Publishing, Co.

CHAPTER 10
THE LATER YEARS AND LOW VISION

Research studies have revealed that visual perceptual training can significantly improve vision as well as reduce age-related health risks such as visual spatial orientation, dark adaptation, visual acuity, depth perception and motion perception and other age related visual risks in the elderly. While the list of age related visual problems is well documented, this research fully outlines the contribution that vision therapy can make to age-related well-being. Considering the impact that aging vision has on accidents both in the home and on the road, this confirms that perceptual visual training should be considered for improving the standard of living of our growing aging population as well as improve the safety of all of us.

The research, funded by a grant from the National Institute on Aging was completed at the University of California and Boston University. Researchers Andersen, Ni, Bower; and Watanabe determined that certain visual therapy tasks have the ability to improve the vision, health and mobility of adults older than 65. Results were published in a 2010 online issue of the *Journal of Vision*. (Anderson, Ni, Bower, Watanabe 2010)

Their results further suggest that the brain changes in the visual cortex, the part of the brain that processes visual information. This research further confirms that there continues to be a high degree of brain plasticity in the both the young and the mature family member and that vision therapy can help all ages.

Older adults often give up too soon and too easily. Because of a visual problem, they may find that they begin to give up on activities that mean a great deal in their lives. Often these are the pleasures they had looked forward to enjoying in retirement. All the books they'd planned to read; now it hurts their eyes to read more than a few pages. All the long, leisurely trips by car now become fear to drive because they can't see well enough and their responses are too slow. Afternoons once spent leisurely on the golf or tennis court turn into challenging times to see the ball, let alone hit it.

Many give up their cherished independence and move into a retirement home of some sort. When residents of a continuing care facility in Pennsylvania were surveyed, failure of vision was one of the most common reasons given for leaving their homes. The eyes lead the body, and because their eyes were failing them they thought they could no longer cope. The tragedy is that in so many cases they give up unnecessarily.

Usually older people have taken their problems to an eye doctor and found out that their prescription is correct and their eyes show no signs of disease. They say that nonetheless their eyes are bothering them. All too often the eye doctor replies with something like: "It can't be helped. It's part of growing old." The second statement is correct. It is indeed part of growing old.

The first statement is demonstrably false. Those older people who are seeking and getting help for the visual problems that come with aging disprove it every day. Unfortunately those who seek help are a small minority of those who need it.

The statistics are convincing. The most common visual problem of older people can be treated, in an otherwise healthy patient, with a success rate of better than 90%. That has been the experience in our practice. It is also what other eye doctors who offer vision therapy for the elderly report.

After vision therapy, the overwhelming majority of our patients can read comfortably for long stretches of time, can see to drive safely, can go on playing golf or tennis. If they have to give up any of these activities, it will not be because of their vision.

But for every patient treated successfully with vision therapy, there are many others who go untreated. These unfortunate older people find their lives diminished and themselves put on the shelf before their time. All because they were told that "It can't be helped. It's part of growing old."

Our eyes do grow old as our bodies age. Along with strictly medical problems, which may or may not be curable, there is a set of visual disorders, which commonly afflict older people. Among their common complaints are the following:

Visually intense close work is hard to do and especially hard to sustain. They can no longer thread a needle. Many say they can no longer read for any length of time. Their eyes tire and get sore, their sight blurs, and they see double. Reading gives them headaches. They skip words, can't follow what they're reading, and forget what they just read. They fall asleep over a book even in the morning when they're well rested. The housewife who used to shop from memory finds that when she is in the store she can no longer remember what she saw when she looked around the kitchen to find out what she needed.

People suddenly become clumsy. They drop dishes, bump into the furniture. When walking, they stumble and sometimes fall, and that fall may break a limb. Such a fall is potentially much more serious for them than it used to be. A fracture that healed in a few weeks when they were in their twenties may take a year or more when they are decades older.

Seeing in shadowed areas is harder now. So is seeing when they enter sudden darkness: it takes longer to find a vacant seat at the movies. Searching with the eyes no longer works as it once did. Especially in an unfamiliar place, it's harder to locate and identify street signs, house numbers, and a bus stop.

Driving becomes chancy. The driver sees less well out of the corner of his eyes, and so he may not notice a car coming at him from the side. His effective peripheral vision has diminished. He may still test adequately, but when his attention is divided, as it is while driving, the peripheral system won't work as it once did.

Driving in the uncertain light of sunset difficult even for young eyes becomes even more so for older ones. And, as one older person who is himself an optometrist observed, twilight seems to come earlier than it used to. The older person's visual reaction time, or the ability to respond promptly to what is seen, becomes slower with age. This is obviously a critical problem when he is driving.

Traveling the roads of an area with a large geriatric population will highlight the troubles of older drivers. Driving in parts of South Florida, for example, is something like crossing a minefield. Here you routinely see cars creeping along a highway at dangerously low speeds and suddenly making left turns from the far right lane. You see also that the car is essential to the lives of many older people. It is the only way they can get out, can get to the store or visit someone; without the car they cannot maintain their independence.

Finally, the aging amateur athlete finds that something has gone wrong. He may say, "My timing is all off now." He can't see to hit the ball properly because he can no longer judge accurately where the ball is. Such are the major symptoms that older people report, the visual problems that cause so many of them to give up activities for which they are otherwise fit, and for which, with help, most of them could again be visually fit.

From our clinical point of view, overwhelmingly their most common visual disorder is what we call convergence insufficiency (CI). It is no exaggeration to say that this disorder reaches epidemic proportions among older people. Its cause lies in the effect of aging on a very subtle aspect of the human visual system.

When we decide to look at something, the brain issues two sets of orders along two separate nervous systems. The voluntary nervous system orders the muscles that move the eyeball to align the eyes to pull the eyes together so that both are fixed on the target. That is convergence. ("Divergence" is asking the eyes to align on a target more distant than the one on which they are now aligned.) At the same time the involuntary nervous system orders the lens of the eye to focus on the target. This takes the form of an order to the ciliary muscle, located in the eye itself, to change the shape of the lens so that it will cast a clear image on the retina. But this is the key to the problem. The second set of orders also spills over to the convergence system as a reinforcing order to the eye muscles. This spill over command is necessary to the successful working of convergence, of pulling in and holding our eyes on the target.

Over a life span the lens gradually stiffens. As it loses its flexibility, the ciliary muscle is no longer able to bring the lens into the shape needed to focus accurately. The stiffening starts as early as our teens but usually does not become apparent until around age forty. That is when we find we no longer can see clearly up close, notably when we are reading. This is when the nearsighted person, who already needs one correction for distance, finds he needs a different correction to see close up. So he starts wearing bifocals.

With the decline in the ability of the lens to focus comes a corresponding decline in the spillover effect, the reinforcing order to the eye muscles to align the eyes on the target. Now the convergence system begins to break down because it cannot do its job without the reinforcing command. (As is usually the case in disorders of vision, there is nothing wrong with the eye muscles themselves; they are just not getting the right commands.)

As a result, the eyes cannot align themselves properly and they cannot sustain alignment, particularly when doing close work. That is why the older person cannot read comfortably for any length of time. (Convergence insufficiency also occurs among the young, notably among school-age children who have trouble reading, but only later in life is it an epidemic.) It is also why older people have trouble judging the distance of a moving object. Our perception of that object depends in part on the contrast between clear and blurred images as it moves in and out of focus. The loss of that contrast, as a result of diminished ability to focus and convergence insufficiency, makes it hard to tell just where that moving object is, whether it be another car or a tennis ball.

The method of treating convergence insufficiency is well known to those of us who offer vision therapy. We first administer a series of diagnostic tests that measure the specifics of the problem. We then start the patient on a course of vision therapy targeted to those specifics. Typically this will include routines in which each eye works alone, in order to equalize their skills; routines in which the two eyes work at the same time but separately, which will eliminate the common problem of the brain rejecting the messages of one eye; and finally routines in which the eyes work together in binocular vision. The purpose of these routines is to strengthen through practice the brain's ability to instruct the convergence system without the help of the focus mechanism. The typical course of treatment consists of a weekly visit of 45 minutes over four to six months, depending on the severity of the problem and the patient's progress.

Our success rate of more than 90% is by clinical measure. That is the percentage of patients whose tests after therapy show that they have overcome this problem. What concerns patients, of course, is not so much our tests as how they feel and how they now can perform in their daily lives. By the measure of satisfaction on the part of patients who tell us their problems have been resolved to their satisfaction, that they have gotten what they came to us for our rate of success is even higher.

In 2010 TL Alvarez (Alvarez 2010) published a study on convergence insufficiency in an adult population. In the study, Alvarez quantified clinical measurements and functional neural changes that are associated with vision therapy.

Visual perception provides a second set of problems for older people. Their ability to process visual information and act efficiently on it diminishes over the years. We see the evidence in the older driver's slowness in responding to what he sees and in a general awkwardness that testifies to poorer coordination between the eyes and the body.

Some decline in visual perception is inevitable in most people as they reach their later years. But older people who restrict their activities make the problem far worse than it need be. Our perceptual system needs constant practice to keep it accurately tuned. We get that practice in the simplest of everyday actions. Every time we reach for an object, every step we take, we are exercising our perception and our visual motor coordination.

Visual decline can be reversed by vision therapy. Here we administer sets of activities designed to rebuild such visual motor skills as eye hand and eye foot coordination. (We should note here with gratitude the work of our colleague Morton Davis, OD, (1986-1987) who showed that it was possible to help older people regain their visual motor skills.)

The overwhelming majority of our patients report after therapy that their perceptual skills have improved in the ways that matter to them in their daily lives. This patient can thread a needle, again. Another can drive safely, again. Still another can drive a nail without hitting a finger.

For many, it means less risk of the fall that could put them in a hospital for many months. For some it means they feel they can continue to live independently. In their various ways patients find themselves resuming activities they had given up doing. Not only does this enrich the quality of their lives, by giving the perceptual system ample practice, it also slows the inevitable decline caused by time. It adds active years to their life span.

There is an enormous unmet need among our growing population of older people. Just how great that need is may be suggested by the response to an article published in the September 1988 *Bulletin of the American Association of Retired Persons*. The message of the article was that older people were not seeking the visual help they needed. The article ended with a note "for more information" which gave the telephone number of the National Center for Vision and Aging. The switchboard was swamped as soon as the article appeared. A month later they were still averaging a hundred calls a day from older people wanting to know where to go for help. And that was only one of the two telephone numbers listed. Great numbers of older people suffer from very severe visual handicaps that are described as "low vision." The term refers to a visual impairment so severe that an ordinary lens cannot correct it.

Such people are truly crippled. Their handicaps are far more debilitating than those we described earlier in this chapter. Many qualify as legally blind. The inability to read is their most common complaint. Some have given up trying; some can read nothing smaller than a tabloid headline. Some cannot recognize a friend across the room. They cannot navigate accurately in their homes, and they are afraid to go out for fear of a fall or a collision. The space in which they can function is small. Their lives are tragically restricted.

It need not be. Most victims of low vision (from 60 to 75%) can, in fact, be helped. Devices exist with which such a patient can make the most of what vision remains to him. In recent years these devices have been made more versatile and effective, and so the aid available to low vision sufferers is that much greater than it was not long ago.

With help, the low vision patient can come a long way, but, unlike the person with convergence insufficiency, he or she cannot come all the way back to normal vision. Today at least, some degree of loss has to be accepted as permanent. Yet within those limits people can make improvements in their vision that will dramatically change the quality of their lives. One woman, for example, is now reading at a rate of 25 words per minute. To a normal reader, that will seem intolerably slow. Not to her: she had gone a dozen years in which she could read nothing at all. For a person who was essentially blind, 25 words a minute is a godsend. Some people with acuity of 20/400 with glasses (20/200 with glasses in your better eye makes you legally blind) have been restored to 20/70 or better. In some states, 20/70 is good enough to qualify for a driver's license. Such people are still handicapped, but their visual grasp of their world is far better than it was.

Low vision takes two general forms. One is lost acuity. The person's sight is so poor that it is beyond correction by a normal lens. The second is loss of visual field. This can be a loss of central or peripheral vision, or one side of the visual field, and can happen to one or both eyes. In contrast to poor acuity in which everything looks blurred or distorted, vision in such cases is completely blank in some areas, but the same as before in the rest. Loss of visual field is usually the result of disease. Some people suffer a stroke so minor that its only evidence is the loss of part of their visual field. Degeneration of the macula, which is located in the middle of the retina, can cause the loss of central vision. Among the consequences are that a person cannot read, watch television, or recognize faces.

The successful use of a low vision device requires a considerable commitment on the part of both the patient and the practitioner who supplies it to him. It's not like getting a new prescription for your glasses. The patient may have to accept the idea of wearing an odd looking device over his eyes. Most important, he has to learn to use the device, and that can take quite a bit of practice and adjustment. This may be particularly true of someone who has not been able to read for a number of years. The device may require new reading habits such as holding the text at an unfamiliar distance from the eyes. In some cases the patient will have to relearn the art of reading, which can take him some months. Some people start with 18-point type. That's THIS SIZE-and with luck work their way gradually down to normal size letters. Some find it hard at first to walk around or pick up familiar objects while using the device; other patients may need far less training. But no one is going to be able to take full advantage of a low vision device without some help in learning how to function with it.

The eye doctor must also make a greater than normal commitment. Not only must he provide training with the device, but also his examination of the patient should be unusually thorough. Under normal circumstances an eye doctor may spend twenty to thirty minutes examining a patient's eyes and prescribing lenses. But choosing the right low vision device means, after the patient's eyes have been examined and his vision tested, learning enough about the patient's routines to understand just how his visual handicap affects his daily life. This will usually take two to four hours spread over two visits.

Failure to meet these requirements is responsible for a large number of unused devices. The person who obtains a device he hasn't learned how to use is almost certain to be frustrated in his attempts to work with it. Very soon the device will go in his top dresser drawer, there to stay. The patient, and too often the eye doctor, will reach the obvious but wrong conclusion: "Nothing can be done." Not that way, it's true.

The most common low vision device is simply glasses with extra strength lenses. The next most common is a magnifier that may be hand held or mounted on a stand. Microscopic and telescopic lenses are highly sophisticated devices. The microscopic device is a two lens system mounted on regular prescription glasses. It dramatically improves the patient's ability to read by magnifying the print so that it can be seen by the healthy part of the eye. The telescopic lens is a miniaturized telescope, also mounted on regular prescription glasses. It has a variable focus that can be adjusted for tasks at both close and distant ranges, such as, for example, reading, watching television, seeing a chalkboard, and recognizing faces. A prism lens can compensate to some extent for loss of visual field by pulling the blocked area into the area where vision remains. If, for example, the right field is lost, the prism will pull into the person's intact central vision what he would normally see to the right. All the devices, not just the aids to reading, require a period of learning and adjustment.

It should be noted that these low-vision devices are useful only in cases where both eyes are severely afflicted. This is because the one good eye, if there is one, will substitute for the afflicted eye and render the device superfluous. Suppose, for example, that a person has 20/1000 sight (virtual blindness) in one eye, and 20/20 in the other. Obviously that person is seeing with the one good eye. A telescopic lens could restore the poorer eye to 20/200, but the patient would continue to rely on the other, better eye without making use of the eye with the new lens. In cases of loss of visual field, the prism lens is useful only when both eyes have suffered a similar loss.

There are also other, nonoptical ways in which the poorly sighted patient's life can be made easier. Many of these have to do with household arrangements. Older people need stronger lighting. Adding vivid color contrast is a great help. A white plate is much more visible on a dark table than on a light colored table. Dials are available that can be read by touch rather than by sight. A growing number of books are published every year in large type editions. There are even oversized playing cards for those who cannot read anything but a headline.

Vision therapy can also help the low vision patient. Loss of sight is likely to leave visual skills in poor shape. A treatment program aimed at repairing those skills can enable him to take full advantage of his low vision device.

Not all people with low vision are elderly. Although most are over sixty, a substantial number of children suffer from these kinds of visual defects. These are the people who as a rule have the most to gain from vision therapy. This is because their low vision dates from their very early years. The older patient who loses vision later in life was able, in his childhood, to develop his visual skills in normal fashion. His skills may now be rusty, but at least he has had them. But the visual defects of most young people date from birth or a disease in infancy. They have never experienced the normal childhood growth of vision. They are doubly handicapped by low vision, and by lack of visual skills. Therapy that gives such patients the visual skills they have never had can greatly increase the use they can make of a low vision device. Such a case was Daniel S.

When Daniel was an infant, doctors told his parents that his optic nerve had been "burned out," and that there was virtually no hope he would ever see well enough to read. The parents, however, refused to accept that verdict. Although Daniel was badly handicapped, he managed to get through school. He learned to read with large type books, but he never read well and avoided reading whenever possible. Anything involving the use of his eyes was very difficult for him.

In his late teens, Daniel was referred to a low vision clinic. There he was fitted with a magnifying device that enabled him to see better for close work. The clinic referred him to us for vision therapy to accompany his new device. We found, not surprisingly, that Daniel was seriously deficient in visual skills. In such perceptual skills as eye-hand coordination, visual memory, and the ability to distinguish figure from ground, he performed at the level of a six-year-old. We could do nothing about his binocular skills because he lacked the physical base on which to build. Accordingly, we concentrated on his perceptual skills.

After a year and a half of therapy Daniel's vision was greatly improved. From the clinical point of view, his perceptual skills had risen in that time from the six year old level to the eleven-year old. That is an enormous gain for someone so handicapped in his vision. Daniel was functioning far more effectively. He completed a course in baking school that, his parents believe, he could not have managed before.

At this writing he is planning to open his own bakery with his parents' help, thus exhibiting a measure of independence that had seemed impossible a year earlier.

With the combination of vision therapy and his low vision device, Daniel is far better able to handle printed material. He reads much more easily and has even taken up crossword puzzles. He sees better even without the device, which is for close work. This has given him much more self-assurance in seemingly simple but once difficult undertakings like walking around town. He rides a bicycle now and even rode a moped on a vacation trip to Bermuda. Daniel's vision will never be completely normal. But therapy plus his low vision device have enabled this once dependent young man to lead a self reliant life.

References

Alvarez TL, Vicci VR, Alkan Y, Kim EH, et al, 2010. *Vision therapy in adults with convergence insufficiency: Clinical and functional magnetic resonance imaging measures. Optom Vis Sci 87:E985-1002.*

Anderson G, Ni R, Bower J, Watanabe T 2010. *Perceptual learning, aging and improved visual performance in early stages of visual processing .J Vis 10: 4. Published online 2010 November 4. doi: 10.1167/10.13.4*

Davis M. 1986-87. *Eidolonic Optometry. Santa Ana, CA: Optometric Extension Program Foundation, Inc. Curriculum II.*

CHAPTER 11
SPORTS AND VISION

Pete Rose and Ted Williams, arguably two of the greatest hitters in baseball had interesting visual skills. When Pete Rose was asked about his extraordinary ability to hit the baseball, he responded, "See the ball, hit the ball."

Similarly, Don Mattingly, formerly of the New York Yankees, said, "I used vision training to improve my hitting. Your hands must go where your eyes tell you. When I see the ball I hit the ball."

Back in the days when he was the American League's outstanding hitter, Ted Williams used to say that he could actually see his bat meet the ball. Many people knowledgeable about eyesight and baseball scoffed at his claim. Nobody could see that well, they said.

Years later, long after his playing days were over, Williams demonstrated his exceptional vision to a skeptical umpire named Ron Luciano. As Luciano recounted the event in his book *The Umpire Strikes Back*, Williams coated a bat with pine tar and began hitting pitches. At each hit he would tell Luciano what part of the ball the bat had met: "one seam," "a quarter-inch off the seam," etc. Each time Luciano checked the ball to see if it was marked with tar where Williams had said he hit it. Williams called five out of seven correctly.

Perhaps one of the most illuminating experiences I had was while working with Pete Peeters (Philadelphia Flyers, Boston Bruins; goaltender and Vezina Award Winner for best goaltender of the year). I asked him what the comparable situation would be in ice hockey, to the Ted Williams story. Peeters replied, "There is none, pitcher throws the ball, Williams watches the ball. Ted Williams swings the bat, hits the ball. For me, I rarely get to see the puck from the time it is hit to the time when I have to make the stop. Part of the other team's offensive strategy is to set up 'screens' to block my vision."

Hitting a baseball is the most difficult visual accomplishment in athletics. In the major leagues the speed of a pitched ball ranges between 70 and 100 miles an hour. If the ball is moving at 80 miles an hour, it will take four-tenths of a second to reach home plate. Swinging the bat takes the professional player two-tenths of a second. That leaves just two-tenths of a second in which the batter must decide on the basis of what he sees whether to swing at the pitch. The hitter must make numerous visual judgments such as speed of the pitch or breaking ball in or out.

While it might seem that few of us need the eyes of Ted Williams in our daily lives, the fact is that we live in a society that makes increasing demands on our vision.

So some measure of his visual abilities would help us to get a promotion, perhaps save a life or write a book, or do something extraordinary; and, on the basic level, just get across the street without being hit by a truck. Some of us also are amateur athletes, and, as we saw in Chapter 9, driving a car calls on many of the visual skills needed in sports.

A wonderful example of the fact that we do not all see or perceive the same way is illustrated in the following story:

Cy Young Award Winner, Roy Halladay, of the Philadelphia Phillies, pitched a perfect game during the 2010 season along with a "no hitter" in the post season a few months later. Halladay was so thrilled that he showered his catcher, Carlos Ruiz, with praise knowing that Ruiz "called the game". Halladay's praise reflected his admiration for Ruiz's ability to make split second adjustments during a game based upon his perception of the hitter. Quoting Halladay: "Ruiz is able to make adjustments during a game based upon what he sees." Halladay continued: " You have your plan; but there are times he goes away from it and it is usually because he saw something. He is usually right.   So impressed with catcher Riuz's work, Halladay presented him with a replica of his 2010 Cy Young Award Trophy.

With a few exceptions like swimming or wrestling, athletics demands a high degree of dynamic visual skill, the ability to see well while either the athlete or another person or an object, or both or all three, is in motion. This is the kind of vision that is not tested in the usual examination where a seated person looks at a chart that is equally motionless. That is static acuity, and testing it does not reveal how well that person would see if either he or the chart were moving.

Until recently even sports professionals tended to accept such a static examination as telling them all they needed to know about an athlete's eyes. Now owners and coaches in growing numbers are insisting on knowing more about the visual skills their players need. Many teams hire vision specialists as consultants to measure athletes' visual skills and suggest training to improve those skills. These consultants also test the visual skills of prospective players the team is considering. They then will look especially for the skills that are most important for that sport. Their information can be vital, for example, to a professional football team deciding whom to choose in the annual draft.

Some athletes who have undergone vision training credit it with making a major difference in their performance on the field. Billy Smith, goalie of the New York Islanders, is one such. Another is Virginia Wade, who gave her eye specialist credit for her Wimbledon victory over Chris Evert. "He speeded up my reflexes and I gained greater effectiveness on the court," she said.

More recently, Arizona Cardinals Wide Receiver, Larry Fitzgerald said, "Optometric vision therapy made a big difference in my life and my career." According to Vince Papale, former Philadelphia Eagles Wide receiver (subject of the Walt Disney movie, *Invincible*), and Bjorn Borg, Ted Williams, Bob Griese, George Brett and Virginia Wade have all given credit to sports vision therapy. Jimmy Connors, tennis professional once stated "sharp vision has played the most crucial role in my success through the years. If you are serious about your game, you can turn to sports vision specialists to help develop fast reliable reaction time with your eyes."

Most sports demand good visual skills, but the requirements differ from sport to sport and often from position to position within a sport. The skills needed differ according to what is happening. In tennis, for example, both player and ball are in motion; in baseball the batter, until he swings, is standing still while the pitched ball is moving; and in golf the player stands still, also until he swings, while the ball is at rest. If we look at each of the visual skills in turn, we will learn more about vision and also perhaps where these skills fit into our own lives, whether or not we are Sunday athletes.

DYNAMIC VISUAL ACUITY

This is the ability to see while you and perhaps what you are looking at are in motion. Imagine trying to read a standard eye chart while you are bouncing on a trampoline, or to read a book while jogging. Many, perhaps most, people will find they do not see nearly as well then as they do when they are sitting in a chair looking at that same chart. Those who still see well while bouncing have vision that is suited especially to sports involving a moving object: a hockey puck, or a ball in baseball, basketball, tennis, and other racquet sports.

Training can improve dynamic acuity. A shortstop who was performing erratically had excellent static sight he tested at above average, 20/15 but poor dynamic acuity. Vision therapy improved his dynamic acuity and his performance on the field. According to Dr. Leon Revien, a sports vision consultant, a group of sandlot baseball players found that their collective batting average improved by seventy two points after vision training, and they only struck out half as often.

EYE-TRACKING

This is the skill that was so highly developed in Ted Williams. Like Williams, Billie Jean King believes she can track the ball until it meets her racquet, at least sometimes. "I swear that sometimes I see it and sometimes I don't," she told us. "When I do, I see the spin of the ball; that's when I'm on top of my game." The player who can follow the ball closer to the point of contact is likelier to hit it well. The player who loses eye contact with the ball early is likely to look away. Then his eyes will lead his head, body, and hands out of position, and he will wonder why he hit that shot so badly. Gary Player, professional golfer spoke about "being in the zone" and stated, "the prime mental stat is only loaned to you, not given to you." Charlie Manuel, manager of the Philadelphia Phillies stated that "early in the spring training, it is more important for my hitters to track the ball."

Most people find it difficult if not uncomfortable to follow the ball to, or close to, the point of contact. There is good reason for this difficulty, for it goes contrary to our daily practice. In most such situations we make a visual judgment, start our motion, and then look away before the action is completed. Imagine, for example, that you are sitting at the dinner table and decide to take a drink of water. You look to locate the glass, start to reach and look away before your hand has actually reached the glass. We do that because it works in ordinary situations like reaching for that motionless glass. But it doesn't work when hitting that fast-moving little ball, and that is when we have to learn to do it differently. This is a skill that can readily be improved with vision therapy.

In a Wall Street Journal Article, Carlos Beltran, of the New York Mets and St. Louis Cardinals, described standing in the batting cage using a pitching like device, which spurted tennis balls at him with speeds up to 130 miles per hour. The balls had colors blocked on them and numbers scribbled on them. They dart and drive like superfast sliders and knuckleballs. If you focus on the rotation of the colors and writing on the ball it helps to recognize different pitches and improve eye tracking. It also improves concentration skills.

Although not many people find it necessary to follow a small round object moving at 100 miles an hour with their eyes, we all need the ability to perform visual tracking as, for example, in moving our eyes to read this page. For an athlete, how he tracks the ball is important. One can follow something visually by moving the eyes alone or by also moving the head. Whenever possible, and this applies to reading as well as to sports, it is better not to move the head because that extra motion tends to throw off the body's balancing system and to disturb visual concentration. "Keep your eye on the ball" is of course the piece of advice most often repeated, and to it we might add: "Keep your head still." If you have any doubts, watch a batter in the box or a tennis player preparing to return serve or a golfer addressing the ball but make sure you watch an excellent player and watch the head.

DEPTH PERCEPTION AND EYE TEAMING

We perceive depth when the slightly different two dimensional images separately received by the two eyes are fused by the brain into a single three dimensional picture. One eye alone cannot perceive depth. We can of course figure out depth from a single image on the basis of what we know: my hand is closer than the horizon, that apple is round. But those are conclusions reached on the basis of knowledge, not vision. Only in the fused image of the two eyes does depth appear in the picture itself.

Nothing is more characteristic of the athletic eye than good depth perception. One study found that varsity athletes had better depth perception than intramural players, while the intramurals did better than those who played no sports. Another study found that better tennis players had better depth perception than less skilled players.

Our hunter ancestors needed depth perception to locate game and avoid enemies, but there is relatively little call for that skill in the close work that is characteristic of modern times. Reading, working at a desk, staring at a computer screen, even watching television are all essentially two dimensional activities. Most sports, by contrast, provide a lot of visual practice in depth perception.

Baseball, basketball, golf, and tennis and the other racquet games are sports in which the ability to judge depth is especially important. A golfer calculating the distance of an approach shot, a basketball player at the foul line, an outfielder preparing to catch a fly ball, a tennis player going to the baseline to retrieve a lob: all are relying on their ability to perceive depth to tell them where the ball is or where it will be. Billie Jean King once wrote that in judging the potential of young tennis players, she considered depth perception more important than eye-hand coordination or speed on the court. King's own style of play, going to the net at every opportunity, is particularly demanding of depth perception and spatial awareness.

In these sports even a small deficit in depth perception can show up in performance. Under the basket Wilt Chamberlain was one of the greatest players of all time, but at the foul line, where depth perception is crucial, his average was chronically poor. He almost invariably overshot the basket, probably because his depth perception was telling him it was a bit farther away than it really was. Chamberlain tried standing behind the foul line, but even that didn't work. His eyes adjusted to the added distance and he continued to overshoot. Tennis players who, unlike King, prefer to stay on the baseline may do so because they lack her ability to perceive depth.

At the other extreme, archery is a sport that, because the archer sights with a single eye, makes no demand on eye teaming. When we studied the visual skills of Olympic hopefuls participating in the National Sports Festival in Syracuse, New York, we found a surprising incidence of strabismus, turned eyes, among members of the United States Olympic archery team. Several archers had one eye, obviously not the eye they sighted with, that turned either in or out. Probably they chose archery because they were comfortable with its visual demands, though they may never have put that thought into words. Certainly they would have been exceedingly uncomfortable (and less successful) playing baseball.

Since standard eye examinations do not test for this skill, many people with poor depth perception may not be aware of what they are, literally, missing. These are leading indications of inadequate perception of depth:

- Misjudging a fly ball
- Poor net play in tennis
- Inaccurate foul shooting in basketball
- Losing sight of the golf ball on its downward flight
- Difficulty judging distance, as, for example, in golf when putting

- Slap or pull hitting in baseball

David H, the editor, went into vision therapy mainly to ease the strain of close work at the desk where he earned his living. He also hoped to improve his tennis game. It was frustrating because no matter how much he played and how many lessons he took; he kept on making the same errors. Instructor after instructor barked at him: "You're too close to the ball!" He didn't really need to be told, for he could feel it in his awkward stance and the way his racquet hit, or mishit, the ball. But neither David nor the instructors knew why he was hitting the ball too close.

He found out when he came to have his vision tested. A standard test called the Brock String (see illustration, p. 107) showed that David's sense of space was misinforming him. It was telling him that things, including a tennis ball, were farther away than they really were. The cause lay in his eye teaming. His eyes had a strong tendency to diverge, so when he tried to bring them together they always joined their images a bit beyond the object he wanted to look at.

In the next four months David took intensive vision therapy. By coincidence, he did not play tennis during those months. Then he had a chance to play daily for a month. His first day on the court he noticed that the world of tennis looked somehow different. He seemed to see the court in greater depth, with more sense of three dimensions. It was an agreeable, sensuous feeling, as if his view of that familiar scene had been deepened and enriched. The ball looked bigger and yellower and fuzzier. It seemed to move more slowly, almost to hang in the air like a fruit waiting to be eaten.

After a few days, David was playing better than he ever had. He could sustain a rally longer. Now he more often experienced that satisfying "this is what it's all about" feeling when his racquet met the ball in what tennis players call the sweet spot. David knows he will not be invited to play at Wimbledon this year or any other. But, in his sixties, he is playing better and enjoying it more. He curses himself less, gives himself more pats on the back. He hadn't planned on Wimbledon anyway. It was very helpful for the athlete to visually warm up before the game. There are a number of different visual drills, which can be incorporated in to the pregame warm up.

EYE-HAND COORDINATION

So far we have been describing skills of vision alone. Eye-hand coordination involves our response to visual information. We are using the familiar term for it, but it would be more accurate to call it "eye body coordination" since much more than the hands are usually at work. Vision, brain, and body are all involved: vision to tell us what is happening out there, brain to decide what to do on the basis of that information, body to carry out the brain's orders.

Joe Montana, San Francisco 49ers, was perhaps the greatest quarterback of all time. After winning the Super bowl XXIV, he stated, "When things are going well you seem to see more clearly. Things slow down and sometimes it looks like my receivers are running in slow motion."

Eye hand coordination is one of the first skills we begin to practice as infants and of course we use it in almost everything we do in our daily rounds. Any sport that makes use of a ball calls for a high degree of eye hand coordination or, in the case of soccer, eye and foot and sometimes head and when Ted William's bat meets the ball we are seeing the ultimate in the split second coordination of vision, brain, and body.

An interesting sidelight here concerns size and skill. Almost everyone who follows sports will agree that today's basketball players would overwhelm their counterparts of, say, fifty years ago. The same is true of football. Not baseball: in this sport most people think that the best players of the past would probably beat today's best, or at least give them a good game. Imagine that this year's all-stars were matched against this team of players active 50 years ago:

> IB: Stan Musial
>
> 2B: Jackie Robinson
>
> 3B: Eddie Matthews
>
> SS: Ernie Banks
>
> OF: Willie Mays, Joe DiMaggio, Ted Williams, Mickey Mantle
>
> C: Roy Campanella

Many baseball watchers would bet on the old timers to win. Why the difference between baseball and the other two sports? Today's football and basketball players would win by virtue of their greater size and speed; athletes are bigger and faster these days. But in hitting a baseball, what matters is not size but eye hand coordination, and that hasn't improved over the years. If today's baseball all stars would lose, it is because they haven't developed their visual skills as well as the old timers did.

The emphasis in "eye hand" should be on the eye, for it is vision that leads the body. Too often the hands are blamed for faults that belong elsewhere. People who drop things repeatedly are called "clumsy," with the implication that their hands are responsible. More likely, the fault lies in the person's vision. The hands, after all, are doing only what they are told to do. Their performance can be no better than the instructions they get from the brain.

Similarly, athletes are said to have "bad hands" when that is not their problem. Blanton Collier, who coached the Cleveland Browns for eight years, wrote: "We discovered that many pass receivers and kick returners would unconsciously look away from the ball a few inches before it hit their hands. Watch the great punt returners and you will see the head pop down as the ball hits their hands.

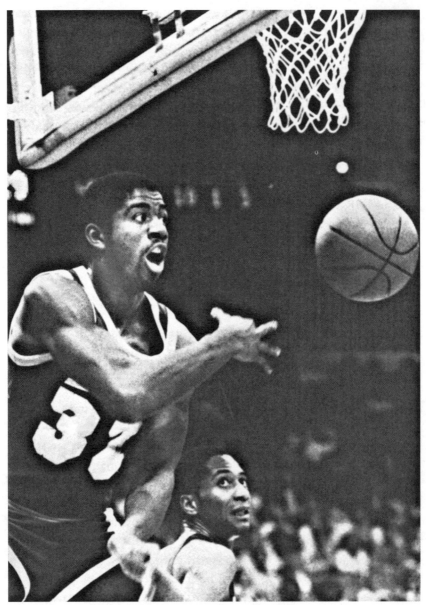

PERIPHERAL VISION

Magic Johnson, former star of the Los Angeles Lakers, passes over his shoulder to a teammate – a play made possible by his outstanding peripheral vision.
UPI Photo

Many receivers, who are said to have poor hands because they muff so many pass receptions, don't have poor hands at all. They simply don't visually follow the ball all the way into their hands." Collier wrote that he was "obsessed with the idea that the proper use of the eyes can improve athletic performance" and that he believed vision specialists should play an important role in advising coaches and players.

"Keep your eyes on the ball" means keep them there until the end, till the ball is caught or hit or kicked. Renaldo "Skeets" Nehemiah, the Olympic gold-medal winning hurdler, found this out when he signed up for professional football and had to learn to catch passes. He was dropping a lot of passes at first. Later Nehemiah told a reporter that his coach had informed him he was taking his eye off the ball before he caught it. "He said, 'Look the ball into your hands. Tuck it away.' I started doing that, I caught a few, and I relaxed."

An oddity of sports vision is that many good baseball hitters have crossed dominance. The dominant eye is the one that leads the eyes in locating the target. Most of us have our dominant hand and eye on the same side, but a few do not. In batting, crossed dominance is an advantage because when a right handed batter stands at the plate his left eye is closer to the pitcher and so in a better position to lead his vision and pick up the target a fraction of a second earlier. (The same is true, in reverse, of the left hander.) If you are wondering which eye is dominant in your own case, here is a simple way to find out. Make a circle with your thumb and forefinger. With both eyes open, center an object in your sight in that circle. Now close each eye in turn. The eye in which that object is still centered in the ring of your fingers is your dominant one.

A very common occurrence often happens when someone learning tennis with a tennis professional. After a number of lessons, the tennis pro says, "You have perfect form, but you can't hit the ball. Voila... eye hand coordination.

PERIPHERAL VISION

We see most clearly in the central field of vision, a restricted zone that extends straight out from the center of the retina. In the much larger surrounding field our sight is not so acute. We see differently in the two zones of sight. In the central field we see objects in sharp detail and not necessarily related to each other. In the larger periphery we do not see detail but instead we see movement and the relationships in space among things and people. In his book *The Ultimate Athlete*, George Leonard called this the difference between seeing with "hard eyes" (central) and "soft eyes" (peripheral).

Like depth perception, peripheral vision is a skill that is little needed in the daily close work that occupies so many of us. A student reading, an accountant totaling figures, a dentist drilling: they are all working entirely in the central field of vision. Our hunter ancestors needed peripheral vision more than most of us do in our modern lives.

Athletes do need it. Most sports, with exceptions like bowling, require good peripheral vision. The pitcher on the mound is concentrating on the batter before him, but he also must be aware without turning his head of the runner on first base. Particularly in doubles, a tennis player must keep her eyes on the ball she is about to hit and at the same time be aware of what her opponents and her partner are doing. Barbara Potter said, "When you're dialed into the ball it's a very central object, and yet you have to have peripheral awareness of where your opponent is in the court.

I call this a feel. I like to have a feel for the opponent, the ball, and my position in relation to those two. All three are crucial, although at some point you can't focus on all three with the same intensity at once."

In baseball the batter uses soft and hard focus to fix his attention as early as possible on the ball. As he waits for the pitch, he holds in peripheral soft focus the pitcher's "release zone" the area within which he knows the pitcher will release the ball. He wants to catch the ball in central hard focus at the very instant of its release, giving himself a vital fraction of a second more in which to judge the pitch and respond.

Basketball is the sport in which we see the most superlative examples of peripheral vision. A great player makes things happen because of his ability to take in everything that is going on all over the court. On some plays it seems as if he has eyes in the back of his head. In the case of Bill Bradley, that was proved almost true. Bradley, the New York Knicks star, and a former United States senator, once had his peripheral vision tested at the request of writer John McPhee. In his book, *A Sense of Where You Are*, McPhee said he made the request after he had noticed Bradley's ability to pass to a man in the open without looking at him.

A Princeton ophthalmologist found that Bradley's peripheral vision exceeded the doctor's definition of the ideal. The most the person with normally good peripheral vision is able to see on a horizontal plane while looking ahead is 180 degrees. Bradley could see across an arc of 195 degrees. On the vertical plane, where the good eye can see 70 degrees, Bradley achieved 75 degrees.

Peripheral vision, like other visual skills, improves with practice and grows rusty with disuse. Young Bill Bradley knew that without being told. He told McPhee that when he was young he used to walk down the street identifying the goods in the store windows he was passing while keeping his eyes straight ahead.

VISUAL REACTION TIME

If eye-hand coordination determines how well we respond to what we see, visual reaction time defines how fast we respond. To an athlete one is as important as the other. Most sports call for both good coordination and quick response.

A hockey goalie is an example of a player whose reaction time is crucial. The puck comes sliding across the ice at 100 miles an hour and often the goalie's view is obstructed so that he does not see the puck till it is almost upon him. The smallest fraction of a second in the goalie's reaction time can make the difference between blocking the puck and letting it through. Similarly, the quarterback's speed in responding when he sees an open receiver will determine whether he gets the pass off or is sacked with the ball still in his hands.

Not all sports require fast visual response. The skill is unimportant in sports like golf and billiards where time is not an immediate factor. On the other hand, driving a car and speed reading are two very different nonathletic activities in which fast visual response is essential.

In tennis the importance of visual response varies with the style of play. A player who goes to the net has less than half as much time as a baseliner to respond when his opponent hits the ball. Bill Drake, Tim Mayotte's coach, has said: "You pick up the ball as soon as the reflexes in your eyes channel it to the brain and start you moving your feet. Obviously, there is variation in individual skills in this area, but I would think that if athletes could be trained to pick up the ball sooner, even if it is a fraction of a second, this would be a magnificent factor toward winning matches."

In fact, athletes, and anyone else, can be trained to pick up the ball sooner. If, for example, you flash a six-digit number on a wall in front of seven athletes for one one-hundredth of a second, only two are likely to identify it. The other five will miss it. But give those five training on the tachistoscope, the instrument that flashes the numbers on the wall, and before long most if not all of them will see what the first two saw. That increased speed will carry over into sports or reading or any other activity.

VISUALIZATION

This most abstract of visual skills takes place entirely in the mind. It is the ability to see in your mind's eye the particular moves you will make in a given situation. You are in fact practicing, for experiments have shown that when you visualize doing something, the muscles involved in that activity respond by contracting. Your body is rehearsing along with your mind.

The value of visualization was demonstrated in a well known study conducted by Alan Richardson with student basketball players. Richardson divided them into three groups. One group was told to practice shooting fouls twenty minutes daily for twenty days. The second group practiced only twice, on the first and twentieth days. The third group, like the second, practiced only twice on the court, but they also spent twenty minutes a day practicing in their heads. In their mind's eye they saw the arc of the ball from when it left their hands till it went through the basket. If it missed, they adjusted their imaginary position and shot till they got it right. The results were surprising. The first group (those who practiced every day) improved by 24%. The second group did not improve at all. And the third group, those who practiced mainly by visualizing, improved by 23%, almost as much as those who practiced daily on the court.

In golf every shot requires visualizing. Before he putted, Ben Hogan would visualize the ball dropping into the cup. Jack Nicklaus describes what he did, "I go to the movies in my head. ...First I see the ball where I want it to finish. . . Next I see the ball going there . . . Finally I see myself making the kind of swing that will turn the first two images into reality." In putting the ball, one of the greatest problems is misalignment. Potts and Roach provide interesting statistics in the published study where they demonstrated that a laser could be used to measure the alignment or misalignment of the putter.

On the value of visualization in tennis, Barbara Potter says: "When I'm visualizing well, I tend to hit the ball better than when I have no image of what I want to do on the next point. On return of serve, I like to visualize placement, as well as the desired spin, whether I hit under the ball or over the ball."

Visualization is essential in a fast moving sport like football. As he waits for a play to start, a good player will visualize in detail what he would do in one or another situation. The point is that once play starts he will not have time to decide how to execute an action. His mind and body must be ready, and so he rehearses them. The fraction of a second he saves may make the difference.

Steve Podborski, former Olympic skier said, "I don't believe any skier could succeed without strong visualization sills." One season Podborski played a game with a reporter where he would visualize and describe a course while he was being timed. He was always within one second of the eventual winning time.

Visualization also serves the purpose of estimating what opposing players will do. By seeing himself in the other person's bodily stance, the player can tell what his opponent can and cannot do from that position, and he can prepare accordingly. If, for example, his visual image tells him the other player cannot easily go to his left, he will prepare for his opponent's going to his right.

Vince Papale, once a great wide receiver for the Philadelphia Eagles, recalls his playing days: "I visualize my pass patterns, how I'm going to get open and make a catch. I can sit here and see myself making the hook pattern, exactly how I'm going to break free. Visualization was also a key for me when I first made the Eagles. They wanted me to run a forty-yard dash. The night before I went onto the starting line, I actually saw myself as a graceful, smooth, fluid animal; not an athlete, not Vince Papale, but like an animal. I just tried to picture being very smooth, very relaxed, and graceful. I went out and I ran a four-five, which was unbelievable for a thirty year old rookie with no professional or college football experience." Recently Walt Disney made the movie *Invincible* (2006) telling the story of Vince Papale. LaDainian Tomlinson, former running back of the San Diego Chargers and New York Jets said, "I always believe you have to envision it before it happens. I have a vision of it happening."

All this is not to say that wishing will make it so. You may imagine yourself stepping up to the service line, racquet back, tossing the ball, and acing your opponent Jimmy Connors! That is obviously not going to happen, nor will that delightful fantasy even improve your game unless you know what you are doing. That is the difference between visualization and fantasy. Visualization is rehearsing, and, just as an actor cannot rehearse lines he does not know, a player cannot rehearse moves he has not learned. The muscles do not know what to practice. Of course, even if you do it right you still won't ace Jimmy Connors but you can improve your serve. You might ace your spouse.

ACCOMMODATION

Accommodation is the ability to change focus from one point to another. When it is discussed in sports, it is always accompanied by a closely related skill, convergence, which is the eyes' ability to align precisely together.

Golf and tennis are two sports that require good accommodation and convergence. In golf, shifting the focus from the pin on the green to the ball in front of you requires instant accommodation. No sport asks more of the accommodative system than billiards. A good pool player focuses and refocuses in three directions: first to the pocket where he wants the ball to go, then to the spot on the cushion where he wants the ball to hit and ricochet, and finally to the tip of his cue. His sight must clear immediately each time he refocuses.

Focusing skills decline with age. The 40-year-old tennis player who says, "I don't know what's wrong but my timing is way off" may be suffering from deteriorating ability to accommodate, which normally occurs with age. So may the golfer whose sight does not clear promptly when he shifts focus from the green to the ball. Middle aged athletes should have their accommodation skills checked periodically. Sometimes convex lenses, usually prescribed for farsightedness, can correct the problem.

VISUAL CONCENTRATION

Concentration follows visualization. It means the ability to focus visual attention during the play itself after we have rehearsed in the mind's eye.

"Concentration in any sport is probably 90 percent visually related," said Mike Schmidt, two-time Most Valuable Player with the Philadelphia Phillies. "Eyesight and preparation are the two most important factors in staying concentrated out on the ball field. By preparation, I mean the pre-game activity I follow to get myself ready for an act out on the field. For example, I may have to mentally prepare myself for catching ground balls on a dirt field instead of on Astroturf. So when my pitcher is warming up, I prepare myself mentally to react to a ball hit my way. When the ball is hit, however, I have to watch it go into my glove. I have to visually react to it; I have to be visually very concentrated."

Concentration is both a state of mind and a visual skill. To illustrate, here is Dave LaPoint of the St. Louis Cardinals describing his pitching against the Milwaukee Brewers in the 1982 World Series: "I got in my bubble of concentration right away. Sometimes you'll hear the crowd, or pick out somebody in the stands. All I saw today was [catcher] Darrel Porter's finger and Darrel Porter's glove. You have to be like that or you won't be around very long."

Centering on a small target helps one to concentrate. Blanton Collier, former Hall of Fame coach of the Cleveland Browns, was the first to advocate centering in football. He told his quarterbacks to aim not at the pass receiver but at some part of his anatomy: chest, shoulder, hip. One of his quarterbacks, Frank Ryan, said: "This target idea is the single most important thing that's ever been told to me but the toughest thing I've ever tried to do. But if you do it, it will improve your efficiency by about ten to 15%." On the other end of the throw, Vince Papale has said that concentrating on the tip instead of the entire football seemed to slow the ball down and increase his chance of catching it.

Bill Bradley applied the same principle to basketball. After setting a record at Princeton by sinking 21 foul shots in a row, Bradley explained that he concentrated not on the basket but on one of the small steel eyelets welded under the rim of the basket.

The idea of concentrating visual attention on a small target is not new. The Mahabharata, the Hindu epic, tells the story of Drona, the master archer, testing the students he has taught. The target for their test is a bird made of straw and cloth hung high in a tree. Drona calls each student in turn. While the first student is taking aim, Drona asks him: "What do you see?" "The tree and the bird, the bow and the arrow, and my arm and you." Drona dismisses him. The same happens to the following students. Then the master archer summons Arjuna, the hero of the epic, and puts the same question: "What do you see?" "A bird." "Describe him to me." "I cannot; I see only his neck." "Send that arrow!" Arjuna's arrow cut the head from the target. He had learned his lesson in visual concentration.

VISION AND THE YOUNG ATHLETE

As we saw in earlier chapters, human vision is not fully developed until the age of ten or eleven and sometimes later. So a game that is visually very demanding, like baseball, will be particularly hard on the youngster whose vision has not completely developed, as is in fact the case with many Little League players.

The visual skills needed in sports are also needed, though in different degree, in the classroom. In Chapter 4 we listed signs of visual disorders that teachers and parents should watch for. In sports, coaches and again, parents should be on the watch for other indications that may signal a disorder in vision. Here are the most common signs, arranged according to the visual skills to which they refer:

EYE TEAMING

- Difficulty catching a fly ball.
- Excessive eye rubbing or blinking.
- Constantly misjudging the distance to the basket. Inability to serve or hit an overhead shot in tennis.

- Frequently running into teammates or opposing players.
- In golf, losing sight of the ball on its downward descent.

ACCOMMODATION

- Seems unduly tired, though in good physical condition.
- Reports blurred vision after practice in school, but not on weekends.
- Reports blurred vision as the school day progresses.
- Has trouble adjusting visually from near to far, or far to near. For example this is similar to those who have trouble copying material to the chalk board from a paper and vice versa.

EYE MOVEMENTS

- Jerky or erratic eye movements.
- Frequent movement of head to follow the ball.
- Inability to hit a baseball.
- Difficulty tracking a tennis ball.
- Inability to head a soccer ball accurately.
- Short attention span.

EYE-HAND COORDINATION

- Poor contact in hitting.
- Player may hit a few home runs but strikes out often.
- Tennis player has good form but makes poor contact with ball.
- Difficulty learning ping-pong, badminton, volleyball.
- Inability to bounce a kickball or basketball more than three times consecutively.
- Trouble playing a simple game of catch: drops ball frequently.

SPORTS PSYCHOLOGY

In closing this chapter, we'd like to mention the area of sports psychology. Roy Halladay, MVP and arguably the best pitcher in baseball, stated that Dr. Harvey Dorfman, sports psychologist, had a big impact on his career. Quoting Halladay, "I don't know where I'd be had I not benefited from working with Dr. Dorfman. I am certain that I never would have had the success I've had, if it weren't for the time I spent with him. It really made a difference and helped me turn the corner professionally." As a young prospect, Halladay said that he was "very distracted by the big picture." Dr. Dorfman increased athletic performance thru his keen insight and by working with the psychological aspects of the athlete.

RECOMMENDED READING

Seiderman A, Schneider S. The Athletic Eye. New York: W.M. Morrow/Hearst, 1983.

CHAPTER 12
OVERLOOKED

Many people don't understand the connection between brain function, vision and personality. Many doctors have trouble imagining these associations, and are quick to dismiss their relationship.

What is important to realize is that all people do not see the world the same way, and that our personal perceptions of the world are not a universal standard. There are many ways of looking at reality and perhaps, many of us who do not struggle with visual disturbances, are the ones who are not seeing the bigger picture. Many people "overlook" the obvious. They "overlook" the research; "overlook" the personal stories; "overlook" basic reasoning skills. Most of all, they "overlook" differences between individual people, and fail to understand that not all people see the world the same way.

This chapter illustrates how perception of the world, through vision, helps construct personality. It is presented as an oral history.

THE CASE OF ANN

Ann is a 58-year-old woman who spent much of her life struggling with health issues, including vision. Ann finally had vision therapy in her late 50s, and she is finding answers to her long-standing health problems.

Two factors played an important role as to why Ann sought vision therapy at her age:

First, she was aware of vision therapy through a personal connection with Dr. Seiderman. In 1989, he gave her a copy of the first edition of his book, *20/20 Is Not Enough*. He was convinced that Ann had vision problems because of several key indicators demonstrated by her everyday habits such as her posture, ways of looking at things, and mannerisms suggesting that she was compensating, that clearly she had untreated vision problems. Simply put, Dr. Seiderman readily identified Ann's binocular and spatial visual problems in the early 1980s. Only after she became seriously ill did she begin to seek professional help.

Second, the onset of chronic fatigue syndrome at age 36 heightened symptoms of a vision problem that resulted in a referral to a neuro-opthalmologist associated with the Chronic Fatigue Center where Ann was receiving treatment. The treatment suggested was to apply paste-on prisms. When Ann asked specifically about vision therapy, the neuro-opthalmologist dangled a pencil in front of her face and remarked, "Oh, you mean this?" The inquiry ended there.

Ann's story is one of a person who spent her life trying to fit in knowing that, somehow, she was different. She was not like others, but had to learn how to "pass" for normal. She had a hard time explaining the differences she felt.

It was a hard road and long way to go in order to get through each day at school. She cleverly crafted work-around strategies just to try to keep up with other students. She was smart, but did not do well in school because she could not concentrate when trying to read. In fact, reading made her dizzy and sick. As a result, the "smart/different" dichotomy was pervasive to the point that she felt like she did not fit in anywhere. Although she was a bright student with a high IQ, she was often in the guidance counselor's office as a highly intelligent, yet low performing student.

In college, Ann continued to have didactic performance problems. She had to study at 4:00 a.m. before she did anything else because it was the only time she could focus. At any other time of the day, she would struggle with heavy eyes occurring only minutes into her studying. She would close her eyes, and then fall asleep. She needed private tutoring for certain subjects. It took Ann 10 years to earn her under-graduate degree from an Ivy League university. She matriculated in 1978, and was graduated in 1988, going part time.

In 1989, when Ann was 36 years old, she experienced a series of flu bouts. After one year with no sign of improvement, a world-renown expert in the field finally diagnosed Ann with chronic fatigue syndrome. During the next several years, she was unable to do anything for more than a half hour without lying down and closing her eyes. The exhaustion simply "put her in bed." She could not listen to music. Sounds, words, and smells ... everything was exhausting. Ann could not walk more than a city block without sitting down to rest. When she tried to read, she would have to lie down, and her legs would actually ache.

In an attempt to address the reading complication, Ann's chronic fatigue physician referred her to a neuro-opthalmologist connected with the Chronic Fatigue Center.

Here is an excerpt from the neuro-opthalmology report found in her medical history:

> *"She is here specifically because of a problem she has when reading and had this problem since February of 1989 and she relates this to a series of bouts of the flu. She describes that the following events occur mostly when she is reading and also when she is doing near tasks. She states that reading disturbs her the most.*

> *She is able to read for a very short period of time. When I asked about a Time Magazine - maybe reading one paragraph or one column, she then begins to feel something that requires her to close her eyes or look away from the page. We talked about this at some length but she is not sure what that visual sensation is or if, in fact, it is a visual sensation. She then feels a "pins and needles sensation" that goes down her body to her legs that necessitates her lying down and putting her feet up. She describes this as a sort of jet lag or*

carsick feeling although not frank vertigo or dizziness, more of a nausea type of symptom.

Because of this reading difficulty and the fact that she had seen a variety of physicians, 22 as a matter of fact, without a diagnosis, she saw a neuro-opthalmologist who did a compete evaluation, including eye movement recordings. He found that she did have convergence insufficiency, and gave her the option of reading glasses with paste-on prisms to overcome the convergence insufficiency. Later in the same report, the neuro-ophthalmologist stated: "Ann's primary symptom is presumed to be visual."

Ann did not find the glasses with paste-on prisms to be helpful, and felt resigned to live with her vision problems, particularly since the neuro-opthalmologist was not an advocate of vision therapy as a viable treatment modality.

Through a friend's encouragement, Ann was reconnected with Dr. Seiderman and finally underwent vision therapy nearly 20 years after being seen by neuro-opthalmology specialists. Now, Ann understands the symptoms of convergence insufficiency and double vision. Before, she could not track while she was reading. For example, when reading one page at a time, she could not read all of the words. She would have to skim the page. She had trouble going from left to right (tracking). In her evaluation it was documented that she was seeing double as far as 24" away from her eyes. We ask the reader to imagine just how tiring and frustrating this may be, not to mention the feeling of anger over having to work so hard to get around this problem of chronic double vision. Ann finally got vision therapy.

As Ann self-reflects, after having vision therapy and experiencing a different view of the world, she admits that vision therapy later in life is a huge challenge. There is a realization that personality is shaped by experience, and to visually experience a new world raises questions about the past. She states that, "there are days you want to put on the old shoe so you don't have to relearn life. Vision therapy later in life makes you realize that you have been living in an alternative world, a world filled with struggle and adaptation. The "new world of vision" after therapy is like a rebirth where you experience new things in ways you could not do with visual insufficiency. Vision therapy was not easy, but its effects are far reaching into making the world easier and better to experience."

Since having vision therapy, Ann knows that her eyes are not supposed to flip all over the page and she can, with effort, get her brain to calm down to do the tracking necessary for efficient reading. Ann now thinks about what people say when they are talking to her. Her double vision has basically disappeared. Her suppression is pretty much disappeared. Ann's visual tracking still remains a challenge but with so many years of delay in getting therapy, she is managing.

We asked how she feels the possibilities in life might be after vision therapy. Ann responds in her own words:

"With the knowledge that there is a connection between brain function, vision and personality, I can find comfort in knowing that vision problems cannot only be recognized and diagnosed, but that vision therapy offers patients holistic noninvasive treatment with decades of scientifically proven successful outcomes. In fact the published literature is robust.

If I had one big wish in life it would be, to not have been overlooked as a kid with vision problems struggling in school. If I had been professionally helped in elementary school, perhaps my name would be on the outside of a book rather than a subject within one, such as this. At least in the 60s, kids like me were called "space cadets" in school, now they are labeled ADD or ADHD and sent home with drugs.

For the readers, I have one last thing I want to say. The way to recovery of a life that was adapted, at least in part as a result of vision disorders, is accepting, with patience, different world views of the believers and the nonbelievers, alike"

In summary, Ann did not see what other people saw. Is this possible? Of course! This is what this book is all about, and why it was written.

CHAPTER 13
FOR A VISUALLY AWARE WORLD

Since the eyes are a bilateral organ, it is not only necessary to have individually healthy eyes, but to have eyes that work well together. Just as legs need messages from the brain to walk or run, the eyes need to coordinate as well. The eyes and brain teach each other form and function throughout life, rehearsing function together during each decade we live. To maximize eye brain coordination is to take our most valued perceptual sense and foster, not just 20/20 eyesight, but aim for full capacity visual awareness. Without good vision we cannot fully take in the world around us nor can we hear, think, speak, comprehend or fully concentrate. Without good vision we can fall short of our potential in life. For all of these reasons, our society needs to have full visual awareness.

Suppose that the society we live in were close to 100% visually aware. Suppose, that is, that we were geared to meet the growing demands on people's vision that we have described in the preceding chapters. This is how that society would differ from the present. Suppose that every school system, from grade school through college, would have its vision consultant. This would not be someone who just checks the eyeballs individually, rather a doctor who understands that the visual requirements of learning go far beyond 20/20.

Today only a minority of schools have such expert advice available to them. The vision consultant would screen children referred to this professional and if visual problems were found, the parents would be immediately informed. Similarly this professional would screen the lowest achievers in the class for visual disorders and also those who appear to be performing below their intellectual potential. He or she would be a member of the evaluation team that advises on class placement and would help determine if a child's visual development is keeping up with the child's chronological age.

Every school nurse will be provided with a simple device with which each child could be screened for visual problems. Such a productive system of educational evaluation does not exist today, but it could easily be designed at minimal cost. Today all that nurse has is a Snellen chart. Every teacher should be able to refer to the nurse for screening any child who is having trouble learning or who shows symptoms of visual problems. If the screening shows there is a visual problem, the child would be referred to the vision consultant.

The result: the 75 percent of learning disabled children who have visual problems would be treated, and treated early in their school history, before the problems seriously derail their experience of education. Early intervention would prevent frustration and loss of confidence at a time when it is most critical. In some cases, the therapy would be enough by itself to put the child back on the path of successful learning. For others, treatment would remove the visual roadblock and so make it possible for the child to benefit from other kinds of help. Children would not be asked to read before they are visually ready.

Vocational guidance would include consideration of vision. This kind of counselor, in concert with the school vision consultant, would suggest to high school students the kinds of career for which their vision is best suited. Students would be warned if they were considering a career in which their vision would prove a handicap.

An example is a student with poor spatial perception who is thinking of taking up architecture. Such students would have the choice between seeking to improve those skills and changing their career plans. The result: fewer young people would go into occupations in which a poorly adapted visual system would hold them back and afflict their lives with stress and unhappiness.

Every young person sent to prison (or other kinds of incarceration) would be screened for visual defects. Every prison rehabilitation program that includes schooling would also include vision treatment. The result: a dramatic drop in the rate of repeat offenses by juveniles; less crime.

Employers would include vision in their plans. Vision consultants would help plan the workspace to minimize visual stress and maximize performance. All those who work with backlit screens would be required to have a visually healthy work environment. Computer users would get a short break every hour. Wellness programs for executives and other desk workers would include vision testing and, if needed, therapy to correct defects or enhance visual skills. Intuitive employers would make such changes voluntarily because they would know that visually healthy workers make for a healthier balance sheet; shortsighted employers would be required to comply. The result: a work force that is more productive because its members are less subject to absenteeism and below-par performance due to visual stress on the job.

Every state's automobile licensing system will require a much more extensive examination for the visual skills needed for safe driving. Here again, a simple device can be produced with which a layperson will screen applicants in no more than four or five minutes. Applicants that fail the test will be encouraged to improve their skills and try again. Students in driver-education courses will be similarly screened. In this case, treatment will be provided for those who need it. No student would pass driver education without the visual skills needed for licensing. Drivers who have reached the age at which visual skills diminish would be screened frequently and required to remedy, if possible, skills they have lost.

The result: fewer visually handicapped drivers, far fewer accidents and deaths on the highways.

Every alcohol and/or drug rehab program will include complete vision evaluation and follow-up therapy programs when so indicated. This will include visual vocational guidance as well. The result will be greater future success for the addict and a higher "cure rate," and, most probably a drop in the country's crime rate.

Every sports team, from Little League to the Olympics, will have its vision consultant. Again, this would be a visually aware practitioner, not an "eyeball person." The Little League consultant would screen out children whose visual systems are still too immature for them to be playing.

In high school and college, the consultant will screen out young people whose visual systems make them particularly prone to injury. At all levels, the consultant will help young people perform better as well as more safely. Consultants to professional teams will show athletes how to minimize risk while maximizing performance. Nowhere is such expert advice so needed as on state boxing commissions. Boxers need frequent visual screening, for a decline in, say, visual reaction time can expose a fighter to ring injuries that will leave him brain-damaged or even cause his death.

The result: better and safer athletic performance, better athletes and far fewer sports injuries all the way from grade school to Super Bowl. Professional schools, beginning with medical schools, whose graduates deal in any way with people's vision, will add to their curricula courses in the development and functioning of vision so that no one will graduate without understanding that vision begins but does not end with the eyeball. In medical school, this is obviously most important in the case of ophthalmologists. The new kind of medical education will produce no more eye doctors who are ignorant of what we have learned about vision in the last 50 years.

It is also essential for pediatricians to understand the role vision plays in early childhood development, and, at the other end of the lifespan, for geriatric specialists to know it is no longer true that "nothing can be done" for older people whose vision has diminished through the natural process of aging. Schools of education will make sure that future teachers know how vision affects the process of learning.

The result: eye doctors will provide for people's visual needs because they do not share the ignorant fatalism of today's practitioners; young children's visual needs will be diagnosed and treated before they confront the demands of school; older people will be able to lead more active and happier lives because they will no longer suffer from unnecessary visual handicaps.

We foresee other changes that will result from people's greater understanding of the needs of human vision. Toy and game manufacturers, for example, will design their products to stimulate visual skills rather than, as is too often the case today, depriving children of the opportunity to learn because the device does the visual tasks for them. Another example is in the design and arrangement of the home. Visually aware parents will arrange an infant's world to stimulate, not restrict, the growth of his visual skills. Builders of geriatric communities will design living spaces in ways that have stronger lighting and color contrast, to name just two things that are most suited to people with aging vision. Many other changes will come as a result of heightened awareness.

Such is our vision of the visually aware society. The cost will be minimal. The payoff will be enormous. The time to start is now.

RESEARCH ON VISION THERAPY

Vision therapy in its many aspects has been the subject of a vast amount of scholarly study with the gold standard research method being the randomized clinical trial. What follows in this third edition, is an updated summary of some of the major research findings on the main topics covered in this book, with references for those who may want to explore the subject still further. What has recently become significant are a number of studies that provide, statistically backed, solid scientific evidence for successful treatment of convergence insufficiency unique to in-office based vision therapy. These studies unequivocally confirm that office based therapy with home reinforcement is the most effective treatment for convergence insufficiency.

As one can see from perusing what follows, there are many references that were published twenty and thirty years ago. These were part of the first and second editions. We chose not to delete these studies because of when they were published, in fact, it is important to leave them here for the reader to know that vision therapy as a profession is not new. The professionals who specialize in vision therapy are expert clinicians who practice the art developmental and behavioral optometry within the broader field of general optometry.

Mitchell Scheiman, OD has published a number of significant studies which further reinforce the scientific facts supporting in-office vision therapy as the best choice of treatment for convergence insufficiency as well as learning related vision problems. He and his colleagues' research studies have been supported by grants from both the NIH (National Institute of Health) as well as the National Eye Institute.

Scheiman M, Cotter S, Mitchell GL, Cooper J, Kulp M. Rouse M, Hertle R, Redford M. Borsting E, London R, Wensveen J, Redford M. and the Convergence Insufficiency Treatment Trial (CITT) Study Group. A Randomized Clinical Trial of Treatments for Convergence Insufficiency in Children. Arch Ophthalmol. 2005;123:14-24.

The objective of this study was to compare vision therapy, pencil push-ups and placebo vision therapy as treatments for symptomatic convergence insufficiency in children ages 9 to 18 years of age. The results overwhelmingly supported in-office vision therapy as more effective than pencil push-ups or placebo therapy.

The CITT referred to above was developed to investigate the best treatment for convergence insufficiency. This gold standard designed study was conducted at several clinical research sites across the United States and was supported by grants from the National Eye Institute, National Institutes of Health, and the Department of Health and Human Services.

In 2011 another evidence based study supporting in-clinic vision therapy was published by Shin, Park and Maples. Shin HS, Park SC, Maples WC. Effectiveness of vision therapy for convergence dysfunctions and long-term stability after vision therapy. Ophthalmic Physiol Opt. 2011;31:180-9. http://www.ncbi.nlm.nih.gov/pubmed/21309805 This study supports the notion that vision therapy is a successful method of treating convergence insufficiency.

VISION AND LEARNING DISABILITY

A number of studies have shown the high correlation between visual disorders and reading problems and other kinds of learning disability. (It should be noted here that these visual disorders do not include refractive error or eye disease. Other studies have shown little or no correlation between those problems and learning disability.)

Harold Solan published a plethora of vision therapy research on reading, reading comprehension, disability and visual processing studies. Solan HA, Shelley-Tremblay JP, Hansen PC, Larson S. Is There a Common Linkage Among Reading Comprehension, Visual Attention, and Magnocellular Processing? J Learn Disabil. 2007;40:270-8. http://www.ncbi.nlm.nih.gov/pubmed/17518218 This study examined the relationships between reading comprehension, visual attention, and magnocellular processing in 42 7th graders. Participants were tested for visual attention skills, cognitive skills and magnocellular processing. The research supports the assertion that there is a relationship between reading comprehension and visual attention.

Other studies of interest published by Solan on reading ability include but are not limited to:

Solan HA, Larson S, Shelley-Tremblay J, Ficarra A, Silverman M. Role of visual attention in cognitive control of oculomotor readiness in students with reading disabilities. Journal of Learning Disabilities. J Learn Disabil. 2001;34:107-18. http://www.ncbi.nlm.nih.gov/pubmed/15497263 This study took a look at eye movement as it relates to comprehension therapy in 6th grade students considered to have learning disabilities. Thirty one students were evaluated, eye movements were analyzed objectively and reading scores were recorded. A brief summary of the results conclude that eye movement therapy did just that and resulted in significant gains in reading comprehension. Due to improved comprehension therapy, there was again improvement both in eye movement efficiency and in reading comprehension. The results support the notion of a cognitive link among visual attention, oculomotor readiness, and reading comprehension.

Solan HA. Hansen PC, Shelley-Tremblay J, Ficarra, A. Coherent motion threshold measurements for M-cell difference for above- and below average readers. Optometry. 200374:727-34. http://www.ncbi.nlm.nih.gov/pubmed/14653660

Solan HA, Shelley-Tremblay J, Ficarra A, Silverman M, Larson S. Effect of attention therapy on reading comprehension. J Learn Disabil. 2003;36:556-63. http://www.ncbi.nlm.nih.gov/pubmed/15493437

Solan HA, Shelley-Tremblay J, Hansen PC, Larson S. M-cell deficit and reading disability: A preliminary study of the effects of temporal vision processing therapy. Optometry. 2004;75:640-50. http://www.ncbi.nlm.nih.gov/pubmed/15508865

The Mayo Clinic also confirmed that convergence insufficiency is a cause of learning disability. (http://www.mayoclinic.com/health/convergence-insufciency/DS01146) (Last accessed 3/15/12) On this website the Mayo Clinic defines convergence insufficiency and goes on to state that when a person has convergence insufficiency, they cannot move their eyes inward together to focus normally. When this happens, it can cause great difficulty reading. This in turn causes parents and teachers to suspect a learning disability instead of an eye disorder. Treatment for this vision disorder can help improve the learning issues. They go on to state that usually convergence insufficiency is diagnosed in school age children.

Another published article expressed concern over statements from other professional associations that seemed to trivialize vision therapy as well as vision problems that may affect learning ability. A review of the references in the statement revealed misleading citations. It seems that evidence-based vision therapy research is often ignored and different treatment options are suggested that may not have sound validity. Based upon these articles there is a concern that professional rivalry may be at the root of unfair judgment regarding vision therapy and the role it can play in reading and learning. Again, vision therapy is not a panacea, but visually related reading problems ought to be considered.

Lack D. Another joint statement regarding learning disabilities, dyslexia, and vision--a rebuttal. Optometry. 2010;81:533-43. Epub 2010 Aug 21. http://www.ncbi.nlm.nih.gov/pubmed/20728412

Atzmon, D., Nemet, P., Ishay, A., Karni, E.: A Randomized Prospective Masked and Matched Comparative Study of Orthoptic Treatment Versus Conventional Reading Tutoring Treatment for Reading Disabilities in 62 Children. Binoc Vis Eye Muscle Surg Qtrly, 1993:91-106.

Seiderman (1980) found that 73% of a learning-disabled population also were deficient in visual skills. Hoffman (1980) examined the vision and visual-perceptual skills of 107 learning-disabled children from 5 to 14 years old. In their vision skills, he found high percentages of the children deficient in the areas tested: binocular coordination (87%), focus ability (64%), focus facility (83%), ocular motor efficiency (94%). In perceptual skills, he found them deficient as follows: bilateral integration (46%), directionality (74%), visual discrimination (50%), figure-ground (53%), visualization (73%), visual-motor integration (81%), auditory perceptual discrimination and integration (44%). These percentages were more than twice as high in each category as the rate found among other children who were patients in the same optometry clinic but were not reported to have learning problems.

Other researchers have studied the relationship between learning disability and particular visual skills. Marcus (1974) found that only four of 60 learning-disabled children scored 70% or more of normal in total binocular efficiency. More important, the study revealed a syndrome of visual deficiency in learning-disabled children. They scored 70% or more of normal in total binocular efficiency. More important, the study revealed a syndrome of visual deficiencies, finding that learning-disabled children suffered from reduced convergence and fusion ability at reading distance, poor focusing flexibility, and poor fixation and eye-tracking skills.

Benton et al. (1972) found 77% of I 15 learning-disabled children deficient in binocular control, and Sherman (1973) reported 92% of a similar population deficient in binocular fusion. In eye-movement skills, Sherman (1973) found 96% of learning-disabled children deficient in ocular-motor efficiency, and Woolf (1969) found 70% to have poor tracking abilities. Pavlidis (1981) found significantly poorer eye-movement patterns among dyslexic children. Beltman et al. (1967) found that 54% of poor readers were unable to follow smoothly a diagonally moving target, compared to 11% of a control group. In the ability to focus, both Sherman (1973) and Woolf (1969) found more than 70% of learning-disabled children deficient.

In the area of perceptual skills, Birch and Belmont (1965) reported that reading readiness correlated more closely with auditory-visual integration than with IQ. Silver (1961) found that nine of 10 children with reading disabilities had deficits in visual perception, especially in figure-ground perception. Other researchers reported figure-ground deficiencies among learning disabled children (Ayres, 1969; Cruikshank, 1967; Eisenberg, 1966; Seiderman, 1972; Silver, 1961; Solan and Seiderman, 1970). In visual directionality, Sherman (1973) and Seiderman (1973) found that 76-78% of learning-disabled children experienced difficulty. Woolf (1960) reported that 60% of a similar population failed a directionality test. In visual-motor skills, Silver and Hagin (1967) reported that 92% of a dyslexic population showed deficits. Sherman (1973) showed a 92% incidence of eye-hand coordination problems among learning-disabled children.

Similar findings have been reported by Ilg and Ames (1966) and Koppitz (1966). Valuable studies in this field, including all those cited above, are:

Atzmon D. Positive effect of improving relative fusional vergence on reading and learning disabilities. Binoc Vis 1985;I:39-43.

Ayres AJ. Deficits in sensory integration in educationally handicapped children. J\ Learn Dis 1969;2:160-68.

Bettman JW, Stern EL, Whitsell LJ, Gofman HE. Cerebral dominance in developmental dyslexia. Arch Ophthalmol 1967;78;722-29.

Benton CD., Jr., McCann JW, Larson MA. Practical approach for the ophthalmologist. J Pediatr Ophthalmol 1972;5:25--9.

Birch HG, Belmont L. Auditory-visual integration, intelligence and reading ability in schoolchildren. Percept Mot Skills 1965;20:295-305.

Cruikshank WM. The brain-injured child in home, school and community. New York: Syracuse University Press, I 967.

Eisenberg L. The management of the hyperkinetic child. Dev Med Child Neurol 1966;8,:593-98.

Forrest E. Visual imagery as an information processing strategy. J Learn Dis 1981; 14:584-86.

Haddad HM, Isaacs NS, Onghena K, et al. The use of orthoptics in dyslexia. J Learn Dis 1984;17:142-144.

Hoffman LG. Incidence of vision difficulties in children with learning disabilities. J Am Optom Assoc 1980;51:447-51.

Ilg F, Ames LB. School Readiness. New York: Harper & Row, 1966.

Koppitz E. The Bender-Gestalt Test for Young Children. New York: Grune & Stratton, 1966.

Ludlam W. Visual electrophysiology and reading/learning difficulties. J Learn Dis 1981;14:587-90.

Marcus S. A syndrome of visual constrictions in the learning-disabled child. J Am Optom Assoc 1974;45:6.

Pavlidis, G. Do eye movements hold the key to dyslexia? Neuropsychologia 1981;19:57-64.

Seiderman AS. A look at perceptual-motor training. Academ Ther 1972;7:315-21.

Seiderman AS. An optometric approach to the diagnosis of visually based problems in learning. In: Gerald Leisman, ed. Basic Visual Processes and Learning Disability. Springfield, Ill.: Charles C. Thomas, 1976.

Seiderman AS. Optometric vision therapy results of a demonstration project with a learning disabled population. J Am Optom Assoc I980;51:489-93.

Seiderman AS. Preliminary findings of a program of optometric vision therapy in an academic environment. Paper presented at the Gesell Institute of Child Development, New Haven, Conn., June 1973.

Seiderman AS. Guest Editor. J Learn Dis 1981;14.

Sherman, A. Relating vision disorders to learning disability. J Am Optom Assoc 1973;44:140-41.

Silver AA. Diagnostic considerations in children with learning disability. Bull Orton Soc 1961;11:91.

Silver AA, Hagin RA. Strategies of intervention in the spectrum of defects in specific reading disability. Bull Orton Soc 1967;11:91.

Solan HA. A rationale for the optometric treatment and management of children with learning disabilities. J Learn Dis 1970;3:635-39.

Wachs H. Visual implications of Piaget's theory of cognitive development. J Learn Dis 1981;14:581-83.

Woolf, D. Dyschriesopia: A syndrome of visual disability. In: Wold RM, ed. Visual and Perceptual Aspects for the Achieving and Underachieving Child.. Seattle: Special Child. Publications, 1969.

THE EFFECT OF VISION THERAPY ON ADHD AND ADD

Learning related vision problems may include difficulty with word or letter reversal, loss of place while reading, short or disconnected attention span, loss of place while reading along with loss of reading concentration and comprehension, frustration while doing close work and most of all under performance. Many of these vision related manifestations are confused or clouded by the criteria used to diagnose attention deficit and hyperactivity disorders.

The relationship between visual problems in school age children and suspicion of ADD/ADHD has been very well documented in the literature over the last two decades. Here are a few prominent studies that may be helpful for the reader seeking additional scholarly work on the topic:

Granet DB, Gomi CF, Ventura R, Miller-Scholte A. The Relationship between Convergence Insufficiency and ADHD. Strabismus 2005 Dec;13:163-8. http://www.ncbi.nlm.nih.gov/pubmed/16361187

Farrar R, Call M, Maples WC. A comparison of the visual symptoms between ADD/ADHD and normal children. Optometry. 2001;72:441-51. http://www.ncbi.nlm.nih.gov/pubmed/11486939 The purpose of this article was to document the visual system symptoms that may coexist with treated ADD or ADHD. According to these authors the current literature indicates that ADD and or ADHD patients may experience visual system dysfunction. The results of the study conclude that children with ADD or ADHD, even with current medical treatment, exhibit more visual and quality of life symptoms than do a similar group of non-ADD/ADHD children.

Rita Rubin discussed the same topic in *USA Today* in 2008. The article, "Sudden Death in Kids, ADHD drugs linked," can be accessed at http://www.usatoday.com/news/health/2009-06-15-fda-adhd_N.htm In her writing, Rubin reports that stimulants used to treat attention deficit disorder increase the risk of death in children who have no underlying heart condition. The drugs commonly used to treat ADD and ADHD have carried warnings since 2006, but she notes that a study published in The American Journal of Psychiatry online estimates that 2.5 million US children take ADHD stimulants according to an editorial that accompanied the study.

Also sited in *USA Today* in 2006 was a news release regarding the new warnings placed on the common drugs used for attention deficit disorder. The report suggests that there were deaths were recorded between 1999 and 2003 and numbered up to 25, 19 of which were children. The report did not cite any one particular drug, but rather claimed that it was a generalized adverse event that was being reported across the full spectrum of drugs within the same class and used to treat ADD/ADHD in children or adults and are in the amphetamine class. These drugs are considered to have a "black-box" warning and sales of this drug have significantly increased over the last few years. This article, "FDA report details 25 ADHD drug deaths," can be accessed at http://www.usatoday.com/news/health/2006-02-09-adhd-drug-deaths_x.htm. In the same week that this report was published, the *New York Times* published an article on the same issue, further identifying these drugs as reason for concern and "black-box" warning.

Laura Novak wrote a widely read article, "Not Autistic or Hyperactive. Just Seeing Double," in the *New York Times* on double vision being mistaken for attention deficit disorders. September 11, 2007 *New York Times*. http://www.nytimes.com/2007/09/11/health/11visi.html Last accessed 7/25/12.

Dr. Eric Borsting and his colleague Dr. Michael Rouse at the Southern California College of Optometry argue that the symptoms of convergence insufficiency such as loss of attention may have a relationship to attention deficit hyperactivity disorder. He observed an overall loss of concentration particularly while reading as well as concentration in class. Failure to complete assignments was a concern as well. Rouse M, MS, Borsting E, Mitchell GL, Kulp MT, Scheiman M, Amster D, Coulter R, Fecho G, Gallaway M and CITT Study Group. Academic Behaviors in Children with Convergence Insufficiency with and without Parent-Reported ADHD. Optom Vis Sci 2009;86:1169–77. http://www.ncbi.nlm.nih.gov/pmc/articles/PMC2888729/ Last accessed 7/25/12.

Atzmon published a very important controlled medical study which showed that the students who had difficulty reading had certain types of eye coordination problems. A commentary followed from Firmon E. Hardenbergh, MD, Chief of Ophthalmology and Ophthalmologist to the Harvard University Health Services in support of orthoptics (vision therapy). Dr. Hardenbergh found the study to be a well planned double blind study. He also felt that the work completed in the study supported the premise that orthoptics which is a form of vision therapy could be appropriately considered for all reading disabled and learning deficient children who have convergence insufficiency or double vision within arms reach and should be considered first in the course of therapy. Atzmon, D., Nemet, P., Ishay, A., Karni, E.: A randomized prospective masked and matched comparative study of orthoptic treatment versus conventional reading tutoring treatment for reading disabilities in 62 children. Atzmon D, Nemet P, Ishay A, Karni E. A randomized prospective masked and matched comparative study of orthoptic treatment versus conventional reading tutoring treatment for reading disabilities in 62 children. Binoc Vis 1993;8(2):91-103.

Meanwhile the Thiagarajan study proposed to show that positive fusional vergence can be trained through a program of orthoptic exercises. Thiagarajan P, Lakshminarayanan V, Bobier WR. Effect of vergence adaptation and positive fusional vergence training on oculomotor parameters. Optom Vis Sci. 2010;87:487-93. http://www.ncbi.nlm.nih.gov/pubmed/20473234 These authors concluded that orthoptics changes the time constant and magnitude of vergence adaptation to BO prisms. This simultaneously results in a reduction of convergence accommodation over time.

It is worth mentioning that Thiagarajan and her colleagues have also received grants from the Department of Defense to study vision therapy and its significance to traumatic brain injury.

Again, it is worth making a note of the Scheiman Study which was also supported by grants from both the NIH (National Institutes of Health) as well as the National Eye Institute reinforcing the scientific facts supporting in-office vision therapy as the best choice of treatment for convergence insufficiency as well as learning related vision problems. Scheiman M, Cotter S, Mitchell GL, Cooper J, Kulp M. Rouse M, Hertle R, Redford M. Borston E, London R, Wensveen J, Redford M. and the Convergence Insufficiency Treatment Trial (CITT) Study Group. A Randomized Clinical Trial of Treatments for Convergence Insufficiency in Children. Arch Ophthalmol. 2005;123:14-24. http://www.ncbi.nlm.nih.gov/pubmed/15642806

Again we can credit Harold Solan for his pioneering work on vision therapy and learning disabilities. Solan HA. Learning-related vision problems: How visual processing affects reading efficiency. Learn Dis 2004;13:25-32.

THE EFFECT OF VISION THERAPY ON AUTISM

Dr. Temple Grandin has authored numerous books and single articles in scholarly journals. In her book, *Thinking in Pictures*, Dr. Grandin explains in her own words what it is like to be a fully functioning productive member of society who personally experiences the daily challenges of autism. Temple Grandin is considered by many to be the most articulate person with autism and has proven to be a major force in helping non-autistic persons, understand the autistic personality better.

She describes growing up as feeling "different." She discusses visual thinking, visual symbols and her cognitive orientation as "thinking in pictures". Dr. Grandin's intelligence and ability to articulate to others the way her visual mind works. *Thinking In Pictures* is a well-documented story about a successful person with autism who has some very special things to say in support of optometric vision therapy.

Grandin T, Barron, S. Unwritten Rules of Social Relationships: Decoding Social Mysteries Through the Unique Perspectives of Autism. Arlington, Texas: Future Horizons, Inc., 2005. In this most informative and highly recommended book, Drs. Grandin and Barron impress upon the reader the challenges of what it takes to live successfully with autism. Starting with the premise that people with autism or Asperger's suffer socially and professionally in their careers because their way of seeing the world is, simply put, different. This difference centers and is articulated in the book as differences in perceptions of the world; differences in how the world is seen and thus on understanding of one's place and personhood within the world spacially, socially and cognitively. It is a most enlightening and thought provoking book based upon personal experience. Dr. Grandin personally supports optometric vision therapy as helpful for others struggling with differing understandings and perceptions of reality and the world in general. It is very well written and for any reader interested in furthering an understanding of how perception effects personality, this book will help to clarify the issue.

Another book authored by Dr. Grandin and very well worth reading in addition to the above book is: *The Way I See It: A Personal Look at Autism and Asperger's*. Arlington, TX: Future Horizons, 2008. In this book, Dr. Grandin addresses autism and its relationship to parents, teachers, and individuals. The spectrum of autism unfolds in many ways and effects daily living. Temple offers helpful do's and don'ts, practical strategies, and try-it-now tips, all based on her "insider" perspective and a great deal of research. Important topics covered include sensory sensitivity, learning issues, unpredictability of the world and different options for medical treatment.

Much of the literature on the autism spectrum and attention spectrum disorders overlap in applicability to the needs of the autistic child or the patient with Aspergers syndrome. The following references ought to prove helpful for those readers seeking additional verification of the valuable role that vision therapy plays in helping these patients in the world they live in:

Eden GF, Stein JF, Wood HM, Wood FB. Differences in eye movements and reading problems in dyslexic and normal children. Vis Res 1994;3410:1345-58. http://www.ncbi.nlm.nih.gov/pubmed/8023443 In this study it was observed that children with language problems, the language problems often coincided with dyslexia. It was found that dyslexic children had significantly worse eye movement stability while looking at small objects as compared to children without dyslexia. Thus it was concluded that eye movement abnormalities had a direct correlation with problems in language.

Another study predicted that children who felt visually confused due to binocular control issues or instability also have problems with language. These authors looks at spelling patterns and found that unstable binocular vision resulted in poor patterns of spelling as contrasted with children's spelling skills who were not struggling with binocular visual insufficiency. The spelling errors that the visually unstable children had were more phonetically plausible than the group of children considered to have normal vision. Cornelissen P, Bradley L, Fowler S, Stein J. What children see effects how they spell. Dev Med Child Neurol 1994;36:716-26. http://www.ncbi.nlm.nih.gov/pubmed/8050625 Riddell PM, Fowler MS, Stein JF. Spacial discrimination in children with poor vergence control. Percept Mot Skills 1990;70(3 Pt 1):707-18. http://www.ncbi.nlm.nih.gov/pubmed/2377403 Dyslexic children were unable to make proper vergence movements when macular sized targets requiring fusion were presented to them. It seems that often dyslexic patients have problems with visual motor control and perception and this may explain the resulting problems they experience when reading.

When children with dyslexia complain about difficulty reading, often they call attention to what they experience and describe as letters or words moving around or swimming on the page. Stein, Riddell and Fowler hypothesized that this is a symptom of immature vergence control which leads to an unstable sense of visual direction. Results of their study indicate that 67% of dyslexic children exhibit poor dynamic control of vergence and that poor vergence produces reduced stereocontrol. Reading improved rapidly (at a rate of 51%) when vergence control is improved. Stein JF, Riddell PM, Fowler MS. Fine binocular control in dyslexic children. Eye (Lond) 1987;1 (Pt 3):433-8. http://www.ncbi.nlm.nih.gov/pubmed/3308532

THE EFFECT OF VISION THERAPY ON READING AND LEARNING

The research literature in this field is enormous. Over the years, but mostly since the mid-1960s, study after study has been published, ranging from individual case reports to research projects covering large numbers of schoolchildren and college students. Here we will cite only surveys that summarize the results of this work. Also the references included in the previous sections amply apply to this section as well.

The first major survey was by Steven B. Greenspan. Research Studies of Visual & Perceptual-Motor Training. Continuing Education Course, vol. 44. Santa Ana, CA: Optometric Extension Program Foundation, 1972.

Greenspan analyzed a total of 111 studies by 80 authors and groups of authors who reported on the effect of vision therapy on reading and learning skills. The number of children or students reported on ranged from fewer than 10 in six studies to more than 50 each in 25 studies. Kindergarten children were investigated in 26 studies, first graders in 28, older elementary schoolchildren in 44, and high school students, college students, and adults in 27 studies.

Greenspan combined the figures given in all the studies and calculated that 72% of the results reported were successful, 15% were unsuccessful, and 13% were successful by some of the criteria used. He then eliminated those studies that he considered flawed in their design or analysis. This yielded these results: 74% successful, 20% unsuccessful, and 6% partially successful.

Since 1974, the *Journal of Optometric Vision Development* has published, usually in its March issue, an "Annual Review of Literature in Developmental Optometry." The authors review papers and research studies ranging in number from 167 to more than 300. Of these, from 25 to 30% are related to vision and its impact on learning and reading.

In its issue for February 1988 (59:95-105), the *Journal of the American Optometric Association* published a special report on "The Efficacy of Optometric Vision Therapy." This report covers 238 papers, of which many are concerned with the efficacy of vision therapy in solving reading and learning problems.

VISION THERAPY AND SPECIFIC DISORDERS

Strabismus was the first visual disorder treated with vision therapy, or orthoptics, as it was then called. Thus it has long been a subject of research. We will limit ourselves here to studies made in recent years, when the techniques in use were largely those practiced today.

All the studies reported functional cure rates of at least 50%. The majority reported success rates over 70%, and for the most prevalent forms of strabismus the rates reported are sometimes over 90%. "Functional cure" means that the patient after therapy has full binocular vision. This is in contrast to "cosmetic cure," which means only that the eyes now appear properly aligned but do not necessarily work together as a team.)

Marcus (1985) reported on the results of vision therapy with 150 patients of ages ranging from 6 years on up. Of these, seventy-six were esotropes (eyes turned in), fifty-nine exotropes (eyes turned out), and fifteen had a vertical imbalance. The overall rate of cure (functional as well as cosmetic) was 76%. Exotropes were most successful, with 88% cured, followed by esotropes, 68%, and verticals, 55%. Thirty-six patients suffered from anomalous retinal correspondence, a disorder which responds much less well to vision therapy than do other forms of strabismus. If they are excluded from the totals, the rates of cure rise to 96% for esotropes, 95% for exotropes, and 88% for verticals.

Marcus found that the highest rate of cure by age, 86%, was with patients nine to twelve years old. For those six to eight, it was 73%; for those thirteen to sixteen, 71%; and for those 17 and over, including adults, the success rate was 70%. Marcus contrasted these results with those of surgery for strabismus. He cited studies of surgery reporting functional cure rates of, respectively, 40%, 11%, and 10%.

Another study reported that 22% of those operated on experienced a cosmetic cure, while 78% were left without effective binocular vision.

In other studies of vision therapy and strabismus, Ludlam (1961) reported functional cures in 73% of 149 patients. In a follow-up study, Ludlam and Kleinman (1965) found that after three to seven years 81% of the patients had maintained their binocular vision, for an overall cure rate of 65%. The rate of cosmetic cure was 96%.

Flax and Duckman (1978), in a survey of research studies involving 489 patients, found a success rate of 86 percent. Etting (1978) found a functional cure rate of 71 percent. If patients suffering from anomalous retinal correspondence are excluded, the rate rises to 89 percent.

Kertesz and Kertesz (1986) reported a 74% rate of success among 57 patients who worked with computer-generated stereo graphics in addition to the usual vision therapy.

Etting G. Strabismus therapy in private practice: Cure rates after treatment of strabismus. J Am Optom Assoc 1978;49;1367-73.

Flax N, Duckman RH. Orthoptic treatment of strabismus. J Am Optom Assoc 1978;49:1353-61.

Kertesz AE, Kertesz J. Wide field stimulation in strabismus. Am J Optom Physiol Opt 1986;63:217-22.

Ludlam WM. Orthoptic treatment of strabismus. Am J Optom Physiol Opt 1961;38:369-88.

Ludlam WM, Kleinman BI. The long-range results of orthoptic treatment of strabismus. Am J Optom Arch Am Acad Optom 1965;42:647-84.

Marcus S. Functional cure rate for strabismus. Research paper presented at optometric congresses in 1985.

CONVERGENCE INSUFFICIENCY

After strabismus, this is the most prevalent disorder of binocular vision. Researchers have reported a high rate of success in treating convergence insufficiency with vision therapy. Cooper and Duckman (1978), in a review of previous research studies, found that 95% of the patients involved "responded favorably" to vision therapy.

Dalziel (1981) reported on one hundred patients who failed a standard measure known as Sheard's criterion. After vision therapy, 84 patients passed the same test. Discomfort and loss of efficiency were reported by 84 patients before the therapy, but only seven afterwards.

Pantano (1982), in a study of 200 patients, found that the majority showed normal visual skills two years after vision therapy for convergence insufficiency. Daum (1984) reported similar results in a retrospective study of 110 patients.

Cooper J, Duckman R. Convergence insufficiency: Incidence, diagnosis and treatment. J Am Optom Assoc 1978;49:673-680.

Dalziel CC. Effect of vision training on patients who fail Sheard's criterion. Am J Optom Physiol Opt 1983;60:982-9

Daum KM. Convergence insufficiency. Am J Optom Physiol Opt 1984;61:16-22.

Pantano R. Orthoptic treatment of convergence insufficiency: a two-year follow-up report. Am Orthop J 1982;32:73-80.

VISION AND JUVENILE DELINQUENCY

Research studies have documented the high incidence of visual problems among juvenile delinquents. Other studies have shown that providing vision therapy to incarcerated juveniles results in a much lower rate of repeat offenses after they are released. The studies are:

Dowis RT. The importance of vision in the prevention of learning disabilities and juvenile delinquency. J Optom Vis Dev 1984;15:20-2.

Dzik D. Vision and the juvenile delinquent. J Am Optom Assoc 1966;37:461-8.

Dzik D. Optometric intervention in the control of juvenile delinquents. J Am Optom Assoc 1975;46:6.

Kaseno S. Screening and treatment program for vision and learning disabilities among juvenile delinquents. Curriculum II, vol. 58, no. 7. Santa Ana, Calif.: Optometric Extension Program Foundation, 1986.

Zaba J, Bachara GH. Learning disabilities and juvenile delinquency: Beyond the correlation. J Learn Dis 1978.

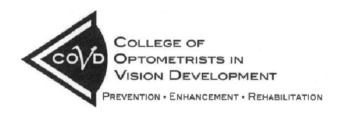

COLLEGE OF
OPTOMETRISTS IN
VISION DEVELOPMENT

PREVENTION • ENHANCEMENT • REHABILITATION

215 West Garfield Rd., Suite 200 Aurora, OH 44202 Ph: 330/995-0718 Fx: 330/995-0719

A SUMMARY OF RESEARCH AND CLINICAL STUDIES ON VISION AND LEARNING

The importance of good vision to reading and learning has been the subject of considerable study. Numerous clinical and research studies have shown that good visual abilities are beneficial to learning to read and to read with understanding. Children with normal eyesight (20/20) can have visual problems which affect how their eyes focus, team together, or move along a line of print when reading.

These learning-related vision problems cause children to struggle unnecessarily, and this can result in their being mislabeled as learning disabled or having Attention Deficit Hyperactivity Disorder (ADHD). Fortunately, effective treatment for these types of vision problems is available through vision therapy.

Vision therapy is an individually prescribed program of procedures used to change and improve visual abilities. Developmental optometrists use vision therapy and special lenses to train the eyes and the brain to work together more effectively. Improvements in visual function enable the child to become a more effective learner.

Vision therapy is a specialized area of optometric care. The following Optometric Clinical Practice Guideline includes a description of the current clinically recognized and supported approaches to the diagnosis and treatment of learning related vision problems: Care of the Patient with Learning Related Vision Problems. St. Louis: American Optometric Association, June 20, 2000

A complete copy of this guideline can be accessed on the American Optometric Association website at www.aoa.org.

A listing of some of the research reports and clinical studies on the relationship of vision to reading and learning ability and the effectiveness of vision therapy in the treatment of learning-related vision problems is provided on the following pages.

STUDIES AND REPORTS ON THE RELATIONSHIP OF VISION TO READING AND LEARNING

Boden C, Brodeur D. Visual processing of verbal and nonverbal stimuli in adolescents with reading disabilities. Journal of Learning Disabilities !999;32: 58-71.

This study investigated whether a group of children with reading disabilities (RD) were slower at processing visual information in general (compared to a group of children of comparable age and a group of children of comparable reading level), or whether their deficit was specific to the written word. Computerized backward masking and temporal integration tasks were used to assess the speed of visual information processing. Stimulus complexity (simple, complex) and type (verbal, nonverbal) were varied. Adolescents with RD demonstrated difficulties in processing rapidly presented verbal and nonverbal visual stimuli, although the effect was magnified when they were processing verbal stimuli. The results of this study suggest that some youth with reading disabilities have visual temporal processing deficits that compound difficulties in processing verbal information during reading.

Bowan M. Learning disabilities, dyslexia, and vision: a subject review: A rebuttal, literature review and commentary. Optometry 2002;73: 553-75, 2002.

In 1998, the American Academy of Pediatrics, the American Academy of Ophthalmology, and the American Association of Pediatric Ophthalmology and Strabismus (AAP/AAO/AAPOS) published a position paper entitled "Learning Disabilities, Dyslexia And Vision: A Subject Review," intended to support their assertion that there is no relationship between learning disabilities, dyslexia, and vision. The paper presents an unsupported opinion that optometrists (by implication) have said that vision problems cause learning disabilities and/or dyslexia and that visual therapy cures the conditions The 1998 position paper follows two very similar and discredited papers published in 1972 and 1981.

This article critically reviews and comments on the many problems of scholarship, the inconsistencies, and the false allegations the position paper presents. Perhaps the foremost problem is that the authoring committee has ignored a veritable mountain of relevant literature that strongly argues against their assertions that vision does not relate to academic performance. The AAP/AAO/AAPOS paper contains errors and internal inconsistencies. Through highly selective reference choices, it misrepresents the great body of evidence from the literature that supports a relationship between visual and perceptual problems as they contribute to classroom difficulties. The 1998 paper should be retracted because of the errors, bias and disinformation it presents.

Eden GF, Stein JF, Wood HM, Wood, FB. Differences in eye movement and reading problems in dyslexic and normal children. Vision Research 1994;34: 1345-58.

It has been suggested that eye movement abnormalities seen in dyslexics are attributable to their language problems. In order to investigate this claim, we studied eye movements in dyslexic children during several non-reading tasks. Dyslexic children were compared to normal and backward readers on measures of fixation, vergence amplitude, saccade and smooth pursuit. The results were compared to the children's phonological ability. Dyslexic children (n = 26) had significantly worse eye movement stability during fixation of small targets than normal children (n = 30). Vergence amplitudes were lower for dyslexics than for controls. A qualitative assessment of saccadic eye movements revealed that dyslexics exhibit fixation instability at the end of saccades. Assessment of smooth pursuit revealed poor smooth pursuit in the dyslexic group, particularly when pursuing a target moving from left to right. Dyslexic children also performed significantly worse than normal children on a test of phonological awareness (Pig Latin). Eye movement results were studied in the light of the findings on phonological awareness: dyslexics with small vergence amplitudes also always have poor phonemic awareness. However, poor fixation control is found in dyslexics with or without poor phonological ability. The backward reading children performed similar to the dyslexics on all tests, suggesting that the deficiencies observed in this study are not specific to children with dyslexia. The problems experienced by the children (revealed by a questionnaire) are in agreement with those measured in terms of eye movement recording sand phonemic awareness. Sex, handedness, IQ or the presence of attention deficit disorder (ADD) did not appear to influence the children's performances on any of the eye movement tasks. The presence of oculomotor abnormalities in a non-reading task strongly suggest that the underlying deficit in the control of eye movements seen in dyslexics is not caused by language problems alone.

Eden G, Stein J, Wood M, Wood F. Verbal and visual problems in reading disability. Journal of Learning Disabilities 1995;28:272-90.

In a preliminary study (Eden, Stein & Wood 1993), we showed that visuospatial and oculomotor tests can be used to differentiate children with reading disabilities from nondisabled children. In the present study, we investigated a larger sample of children to see if these findings held true. Using 93 children from the Bowman Gray Learning Disability Project (mean age = 11.3 years: 54 boys, 39 girls), we compared the phonological and visuospatial abilities of nondisabled children (children whose reading at fifth grade rated a Woodcock-Johnson reading standardized score between 85 and 115), and children with reading disability (whose reading standardized score was below 85 on the Woodcock-Johnson). In addition to performing poorly on verbal tests, the children with reading disability were significantly worse than nondisabled children at many visual and eye- movement tasks.

A high proportion of the variance (68%) in reading ability of both the nondisabled children and those with reading disability could be predicted by combining visual and phonological scores in a multiple regression. These results provide further support for the hypothesis that reading disability may, to some extent, result from dysfunction of the visual and oculomotor systems.

Grisham D, Sheppard M, Tran W. Visual symptoms and reading performance. Optometry and Vision Science 1993;70:384-91.

Clinical observation indicates that visual asthenopic symptoms are frequently associated with reading for long periods of time. We investigated the relation between visual symptoms and standard measures of reading performance in 78 university students. The number of asthenopic complaints increased during the reading phase of the experiment and decreased during the relaxation phase. Overall, a weak but significant negative correlation was found between number of symptoms and reading rate on the Nelson-Denny reading test. The most symptomatic subjects scored lower on vocabulary and comprehension than the least asthenopic subjects. A limited retrospective analysis revealed no reading performance differences between subjects having normal binocular vision and those showing a minimum binocular dysfunction; however, the dysfunctional subjects reported more visual symptoms. This study suggests that visual symptoms are a factor in reducing reading performance, particularly in very symptomatic individuals.

Johnson RA, Zaba JN. The visual screening of adjudicated adolescents. Journal of Behavioral Optometry 1999;10:13-17.

The New York State Optometric Association Vision Screening Battery (NYOSA) and the Developmental Eye Movement Test (DEM) were administered to 50 adjudicated adolescents in order to isolate which particular visual factors are most responsible for the learning difficulties of juvenile offenders. The most significant finding was the high failure rate of juvenile offenders on both tracking tests. Forty-eight percent failed the tracking subtest of the NYSOA. Sixty-eight percent failed one or more of the DEM subtests.

Although adjudicated juveniles have received various psychological, educational, and vocational treatments most of these treatments have had limited effectiveness. It is difficult for a treatment program, particularly an academic one, to be effective if the adolescent lacks adequate visual skills. Unless at-risk adolescents with visual impairments are properly diagnosed and treated, many offenders, such as those in the current study, may end up in the criminal justice system.

Maples WC. Visual factors that significantly impact academic performance. Optometry 2003;74:35-39.

Both race and socio-economic status are correlated to performance in the classroom. Theses two factors are inter-related, since minorities, proportion-wise, are more highly represented in the lower socio-economic strata. Inefficient visual skills have been shown to be more prevalent among minority groups and in low socio-economic groups. These inefficient visual skills impact the students' learning. This study was undertaken to discover the visual skills that were significantly correlated with academic performance problems.

A total of 2,659 examinations on 540 children were administered over three consecutive school years. Socio-economic, racial and standardized academic performance data (Iowa Test of Basic Skills – ITBS) were furnished by the families and the school system. The visual and demographic data from the examinations were then compared to performance on the 21 subtests of the ITBS.

Some visual factors were found to be much better predictors of scores on the ITBS than either race or socio-economic status. Even though the significance of these two demographic variables was small, race and socio-economic variables were each significant in about a third of the 21 ITBS scores. Visual factors are significantly better predictors of academic success as measured by the ITBS than is race or socio-economics. Visual motor activities are better predictors of ITBS scores than are binocularity or accommodation. These latter skills were significant predictors also, but to a lesser degree.

Simons H, Grisham JD. Binocular anomalies and reading problems. Journal of the American Optometric Association 1987;58:578-87.

This paper reviews and evaluates the research literature on the relationship of binocular anomalies to reading problems. The weight of the evidence supports a positive relationship between certain binocular anomalies and reading problems. The evidence is positive for exophoria at near, fusional vergence reserves, aniseikonia, anisometropia, convergence insufficiency, and fixation disparity. There is some weak positive evidence for esophoria at near and mixed evidence on lateral phorias at distance is negative.

Taylor Kulp M, Schmidt P. The relation of clinical saccadic eye movement testing to reading in kindergartners and first graders. Optometry and Vision Science 1997 ;74:37-42.

The relation between psychometric eye movement scores and reading skill was studied in a masked investigation with 181 kindergartners and first graders (mean age 6.25 years) from a middle class, suburban, elementary school near Cleveland, Ohio. Eye movements were evaluated with the New York State Optometric Association King-Devick and the Developmental Eye Movement tests. Digit Knowledge was assessed with Reversals Frequency Test Execution Subtest (Gardner). Reading performance was measured with Metropolitan Achievement Test 6 (MAT6) Reading Test and teacher's assessments. The number of unknown or reversed numbers on Gardner was significantly related to test times on the NYSOA K-D and DEM, but not the DEM ratio. Outcome on NYSOA K-D, determined by errors in conjunction with test time, was significantly related to reading ability in 5-year-olds, 6-year-olds, and the entire subject group when controlling for age. Our findings suggest that performance of the NYSOA K-D is related to reading performance in 5-and 6-year-olds in kindergarten.

Taylor Kulp M, Schmidt P. Visual predictors of reading performance in kindergarten and first grade children. Optometry and Vision Science 1996;73:255-62.

A masked investigation of the relation between performance on various vision tests and reading was conducted with 90 kindergartners (mean age 5.73 years) and 91 first graders (mean age 6.76 years) from a middle class, suburban, elementary school near Cleveland, Ohio.

The results revealed that accommodative facility was predictive of successful reading performance in 7-year-olds, first graders and the entire subject group when age or grade was controlled. Failure on the MCT was significantly associated with decreased reading skill in 5-year-olds. In addition, stereoacuity worse than 100 sec arc, MCT failure plus stereoacuity worse than 50 sec arc and accommodative ability were predictive of whether children of average intelligence would show successful or unsuccessful reading ability.

Thus, visual performance was significantly related to reading performance even in children of average intelligence when IQ was partially controlled. Also, the predictive value of the MCT for reading achievement could be improved by the addition of a referral criterion for stereoacuity. This would make the results of MCT screening more readily applicable to educators.

Taylor Kulp M, Edwards K, Mitchell L. Is visual memory predictive of below-average academic achievement in second through fourth graders? Optometry and Vision Science 2002;79:431-34.

A masked investigation of the relation between visual memory and academics was performed in 155 second through fourth-grade children (mean age= 8.83 years). Visual memory ability was assessed with the Test of Visual Perceptual Skills visual memory subtest. The school administered the Otis-Lennon School Ability Test and Stanford Achievement Test. Age and verbal ability were controlled in all regression analyses.

Visual memory score was significantly predictive of below-average word decoding, total math score, and Stanford complete battery score. Visual memory score showed a positive trend in predicting reading comprehension related to below-average reading decoding, math, and overall academic achievement (as measured by the Stanford Achievement Test) in second-through fourth-grade children, while controlling for age and verbal ability.

Taylor Kulp M. Relationship between visual motor integration skill and academic performance in kindergarten through third grade. Optometry and Vision Science 1999;76:159-63.

The objective of this study was to examine the relationship between visual motor integration skill and academic performance in kindergarten through third grade. One hundred ninety-one (n = 191) children in kindergarten through third grade (mean age = 7.78 years; 52% male) from an upper-middle class, suburban primarily Caucasian, elementary school near Cleveland, Ohio were included in this investigation. Visual analysis and visual motor integration skill were assessed with the Beery Developmental Test of Visual Motor Integration (VMI) long form. The relationship between performance on the VMI and teachers' ratings of academic achievement was analyzed. The children's regular classroom teachers rated the children with respect to reading, math, and writing ability. Second and third grade children (N = 98) were also rated on spelling ability. Only experienced teachers were included in the investigation and the validity of the teachers' ratings was substantiated by significant correlations with standardized test scores. Teachers were masked to performance on the VMI until the rating was completed. The Stanford Diagnostic Reading test, 4th edition, was also used as a measure of reading ability in the first graders and the Otis-Lennon school Ability test (OLSAT), 6th edition, was also used as a measure of school-related cognitive ability in second graders.

Performance on the VMI was found to be significantly related to teachers' ratings of the children's reading, math, writing, and spelling ability. An analysis by age group revealed that performance on the VMI was significantly correlated with reading achievement ratings in the 7- 8- and 9-year-olds. VMI scores were also significantly related to performance on the Stanford Reading Test in the first graders and to performance on the OLSAT in the second graders. In order to partially control for mathematical ability, an additional analysis was performed with children who were identified by the OLSAT as having either below average, average or above average verbal reasoning scores ability (the verbal reasoning score consists of aural and arithmetic reasoning). This analysis again revealed a significant correlation between the VMI and teachers' achievement ratings in math. Finally, in order to partially control for cognitive ability related to writing, an additional analysis was performed with children who were identified by the OLSAT as having either below average, average or above average nonverbal cluster OLSAT scores. This analysis again revealed a significant correlation between the VMI and teachers' achievement ratings in writing (p=0.001 among average second grade students). *Conclusion:* Performance on a visual analysis and visual motor integration task is significantly related to academic performance in 7- 8- and 9- year olds.

Taylor Kulp M, Schmidt P. Effect of oculomotor and other visual skills on reading performance: A literature review. Optometry and Vision Science 1996;73:283-92.

Reading disability is a multifaceted problem, which requires an interdisciplinary approach. Many visual difficulties have been shown to be related to reading ability. Efficient reading requires accurate eye movements and continuous integration of the information obtained from each fixation by the brain. A relation between oculomotor efficiency and reading skill has been shown in the literature. Frequently, these visual difficulties can be treated successfully with vision therapy.

Young B, Collier-Gary K, Schwing S. Visual factors: A primary cause of failure in beginning reading. Journal of Optometric Vision Development 1994;32:58-71.

In a longitudinal study of 144 *beginning* readers in public school, data on 25 measures of visual efficiency were subjected to two-and three-way Analyses of Variance. Binocular function, visual acuity, discrepancies in acuity, and color deficiencies were all found to be statistically significant in impeding beginning reading. Significant differences were also found in the sequence of visual development between sexes, between eye and dominance for different tasks, between specific factors for 6-, 7-, and 8-year-olds and first and second grades. It was concluded that visual factors are a *primary* cause of beginning reading failure and that most current school screenings are inadequate in scope and rigor.

STUDIES THAT EVALUATE THE IMPACT OF VISION THERAPY ON READING AND LEARNING ABILITY

Atzmon D, Nemet P, Ishay A, Karni E. A randomized prospective masked and matched comparative study of orthoptic treatment versus conventional reading tutoring treatment for reading disabilities in 62 Children. Binocular Vision and Eye Muscle Surgery Quarterly 1993;8:91-106.

Schools need better and economical methods of treating reading disabilities. Controversies remain whether orthoptics and/or "visual training" can remedy reading disabilities. Therefore, and to extend our prior studies, we undertook a comparative and controlled study.

120 children with reading disability were tested extensively, matched and randomly divided into three groups: orthoptic, conventional (reading tutoring) and no-treatment control. Unfortunately, participants in the control group were unable to adhere to no treatment and were deleted. Each of the 40 children in the first two groups had 40 sessions, 20 minutes daily. Orthoptic treatment was directed to markedly

increase fusional convergence amplitudes for both near and distance to 60Δ The two treatments were also carefully matched in time and effort.

Examination of subjects revealed that 100% had poor fusional convergence amplitudes by our standards and 60% had 20Δ or less: two-thirds had a normal near point of convergence of 5 cm or less; many had a subjective reading and asthenopic symptoms in the presence of fusional convergence amplitudes said to be normal by other authorities.

Sixty-two children in 31 matched pairs completed the course of treatment and testing. The results were: equal and statistically significant (P<.05) marked improvement in reading performance in both treatment groups on essentially all tests.

Orthoptic treatment, to increase convergence amplitudes to 60Δ is as effective as conventional in-school reading tutoring treatment of reading disabilities. An advantage of orthopic treatment was that subjective reading and asthenopic symptoms virtually disappeared after orthoptics. We recommend orthoptic treatment as: 1) an effective alternate primary treatment: 2) adjunctive treatment for those who do not respond well to standard treatment: and 3) as primary treatment in any case with asthenopic symptoms of/or convergence inadequacy.

Fischer B, Hartnegg K.. Effects of visual training on saccade control in dyslexia. Perception 2000;29:531-42.

This study reports the effects of daily practice of three visual tasks on the saccadic performance of the 85 dyslexic children in the age range of 8 to 15 years. The children were selected from among other dyslexics because they showed deficits in their eye-movement control, especially in fixation stability and/or voluntary saccade control. The eye movements were measured in an overlap prosaccade and a gap antisaccade task before and after the training. The three tasks used for the training included a fixation, a saccade, and a distractor condition. In any of these tasks, the subject had to detect the last orientation of a small pattern which rapidly changed its orientation between up, down, right, and left, before it disappeared after some time. The task was to press one of four keys corresponding to the last orientation. The visual pattern was presented on and LCD display of a small handheld instrument given to the children for daily used at home. The results indicate that daily practice improved not only the perceptual capacity, but also the voluntary saccade control, within 3 to 8 weeks. After the training, the group of dyslexics was no longer statistically different from the control group.

Halliwell J, Solan H. The Effect of a supplemental perceptual training program on reading achievement. Exceptional Children 19972;38: 613-22.

At the beginning of the first grade, 105 students designated as potential reading problems were divided into three groups of 35 children each: experimental I, which received supplementary perceptual training in addition to the regular reading program; experimental II, which received traditional supplementary reading instruction in addition to the regular reading program; and the control group, which received no supplementary instruction. The Metropolitan Achievement Test (MAT) was administered at the end of May. The statistical analysis of the data indicated that, of all the groups, only the experiment I total group and the experimental I boys read significantly better than the respective control groups on the reading subtest of the MAT.

Harris P. Learning-related visual problems in Baltimore City: A Long-Term Program. Journal of Optometric Vision Development 2002;33:75-115.

A longitudinal, single-masked, random sample study of children at a Baltimore City Public Elementary school documents the prevalence of learning-related visual problems in the inner city of Baltimore and tests the effectiveness of vision therapy. Vision therapy was provided to one of the randomly selected groups and data were collected on optometric tests, visual performance tests, and standardized achievement tests before and after treatment was provided. Data presented show that the vision therapy program has made a significant difference in the demand level of reading that could be read for understanding, in math achievement on standardized testing, and in reading scores on standardized testing, as well as on infrared eye-movement Visagraph recordings, which show significant changes on nearly all mechanical aspects of the reading process.

McKane F, et al. A comparison of auditory/ language therapy with school visual support procedures in a public school setting. Journal of Optometric Vision Development 2001;32:83-92.

Some hold that poor reading eye movements are caused by poor language skills and if the auditory/ language skills were improved that reading and eye movements during reading would also improve. Twenty-nine third grade children who had previously been identified as being below average in some academic area were the subjects of this study. The experimental group contained 18 subjects, equally distributed between genders. After screening evaluations, all children were enrolled in an auditory/language enrichment program and the experimental group also received school based vision techniques which were individually programmed and administered by school personnel, in the school setting daily for 30 minutes a day for 3.5 months. Both groups improved significantly over pre-test scores on the reading aspect of the WRAT and reading rate with comprehension as measured by the –Visagraph. The experimental group also demonstrated a significant improvement in reading eye movements as measured by the Visagraph, but the control group did not. The authors concluded that both visual and auditory/language intervention has a positive effect on the reading WRAT scores as well as the reading rate with comprehension. Reading eye movements, however, were significantly improved only with visual intervention and not with auditory/language therapy.

Orfield A, Basa F, Yun J. Vision problems of children in poverty in an urban school clinic: Their epidemic numbers, impact on learning, and approaches to remediation. Journal of Optometric Vision Development 2001;32:114-41.

The Mather School pilot study explores the relationship between vision and learning by analyzing clinical vision data gathered in an urban school eye clinic from fall 1993 to spring 1999, and relating the vision findings with available standardized test scores and teacher grades. There were 1544 vision evaluations on 801 students, 226 extended functional vision exams on students who failed the initial evaluation, 79 children who received some vision therapy and 116 who received glasses, mostly for close work, and another 85 who received prescription for glasses. Our in-school evaluations found a higher incidence of vision problems than reported in previous studied. Without counting the visual tracking test, 41% failed: adding the tracking test, 53% failed. The majority of the vision problems we found were related to near vision, including a great deal of hyperopia, and were associated with lower average test scores. Our treatments of reading glasses and vision therapy improved visual function on specific tests, with those who had the poorest findings on individual measures improving the most. Correlated with these treatments are improvements in teacher grades, percentiles, and grade equivalents on standardized tests in reading and mathematics. Even with our limited study, the data suggests that there is a high incidence of these problems, that some of these problems are correlated with lower scores in reading and math, that they can be treated in a school setting, that school screenings should be expanded to include more near point tests, that detailed functional vision exams should be required of all children falling behind in school, and that The Developmental Eye Movement test, which 24.5% of the children failed, is an excellent predictor of a significant percent of reading failure risk and should be administered to all school children in the early grades so that help can be given early. Remediation for poor visual skills is as important as remediation for learning failure, because lack of many of these skills correlate with learning problems.

Rounds BB, Manley CW, Norris RH. The effect of oculomotor training on reading efficiency. Journal of American Optometric Association 1991;62:92-99.

The purpose of this study was to record and measure, by means of a microcomputer, the reading eye movements and reading efficiency of a sample of "poor readers" from an adult, professional school population. A program of oculomotor skill enhancement training was given to 10 students who also failed the reading test, but received no such training. All subjects' eye movements were monitored and recorded individually while reading, using a Visagraph eye-Movement Recording System. The subjects were split into and experimental group (Receiving training) and a control group (receiving no training). Following a 12-hour program of "in office" and "home" training, the group receiving oculomotor training showed trends toward improved reading eye movement efficiency (number of regressions, number of fixations and span of recognition), compared to that of the untrained group.

Seiderman A. Optometric vision therapy- results of a demonstration project with a learning disabled population. Journal of American Optometric Association 1980;51:489-92.

Thirty-six children attending a private school for learning disabled children were diagnosed as having visual and /or perceptual disorders. The experimental group received individual programming in visual and perceptual development at their appropriate developmental levels. The control group received instruction in physical education, art or music classes. Both groups received individualized reading assistance. Statistical analysis of the two year demonstration project, which included nine months of actual training, indicated that the experimental group made significant gains in reading as compared to the control group. The improvement in basic instructional level of The Informal Reading Inventory (Temple University), and the Word Reading and Paragraph Meaning subtests of the Stanford Achievement Tests, and the actual classroom reading levels were all statistically significant. The Informal Word Recognition Invention (Daniels) and the spelling subtest of the Stanford Achievement Tests showed a definite trend approaching statistical significance.

Sigler G, Wylie T. The effect of vision therapy on reading rate: A pilot study. Journal of Behavioral Optometry 1994;5:99-102.

Three subjects, two aged 8 and one age 10, with identified visual system disorders were selected as subjects to evaluate the effects of vision therapy on reading efficiency as measured by reading rate. Reading rate measures were taken prior to initiation, at the conclusion, and 90 days post-visual therapy. The results were that all subjects had accelerated reading rate gains during the period of vision therapy and that the reading rates for two of the three subjects continued to increase in the post-therapy (maintenance) period. All three subjects experienced positive gains over the period (180 days) of the study.

Solan H, Shelley-Tremblay J, et al. Effect of Attention Therapy on Reading Comprehension. Journal of Learning Disabilities 2003;36:556-63.

This study quantified the influence of visual attention therapy on the reading comprehension of Grade 6 children with moderate reading disabilities (RD) in the absence of specific reading remediation. Thirty students with below-average reading scores were identified using standardized reading comprehension tests. Fifteen children were placed randomly in the experimental group and 15 in the control group. The Attention Battery of the *Cognitive Assessment System* was administered to all participants. The experimental group received 12 one-hour sessions of individually monitored, computer-based attention therapy programs; the control group received no therapy during their 12-week period. Each group was retested on attention and reading comprehension measures. In order to stimulate selective and sustained visual attention, the vision therapy stressed various aspects of arousal, activation, and vigilance. At the completion of attention therapy, the mean standard attention and reading comprehension scores of the experimental group had improved significantly. The control group, however, showed no significant improvement in reading comprehension scores after 12 weeks. Although uncertainties still exist, this investigation supports the notion that visual attention is malleable that the attention therapy has significant effect on reading comprehension in this often neglected population.

Solan H, Larson S, Shelley-Tremblay J, Ficarra A, Silverman M. Role of visual attention in cognitive control of oculomotor readiness in students with reading disabilities. Journal of Learning Disabilities 2001;34:107-18.

This study investigated eye movement and comprehension therapy in Grade 6 children with reading disabilities (RD). Both order of therapy and type of therapy were examined. Furthermore, the implications of visual attention in ameliorating reading disability are discussed. Thirty-one students with RD were identified using standardized reading comprehension tests. Eye movements were analyzed objectively using an infared recording device. Reading scores of participating children were 0.5 to 1 SD below the national mean. Testing took place before the start of therapy (T1) and was repeated after 12 weeks (T2) and 24 weeks (T3) of therapy. One group of students had eye movement therapy first, followed by comprehension therapy; in the other group, the order was reversed. Data were evaluated using a repeated measures MANOVA and post hoc tests. At T1, mean reading grade was 2 years below grade level, and eye movement scores were at about Grade 2 level. Mean growth in reading comprehension for the total sample was 2.6 years at T3: equally significant improvement was measured in eye movements. Learning rate in reading comprehension improved from 60% (T1) to 400% (t3). Although within group differences were statistically significant at T2 and T3. Eye movement therapy improved eye movements and also resulted in significant gains in reading comprehension. Comprehension therapy likewise produced improvement both in eye movement efficiency and in reading comprehension. The results support the notion of a cognitive link among visual attention, oculomotor readiness, and reading comprehension

Sterner B, Abrahamsson M, Sjöström A. Accommodative facility training with a long term follow up in a sample of school aged children showing accommodative dysfunction. Documenta Ophthalmologica 1999;99:93-101.

The primary aim of this project was to study the effect of flip lens-training on the accommodative function in a group of children with accommodative dysfunction and subjective symptoms such as asthenopia, headache, blurred vision, and avoidance of near activity. We also wanted to measure the accommodative facility among the children in comparison with a control group. Another aim of the study was whether flip lens-training increased accommodative facility, and to find out if it also had a positive effect on their asthenopia and related problems also in long term. Following the training period the accommodative facility and accommodative function significantly increased and two years after finishing the training period no child had regained any subjective symptoms and the objective findings were almost the same as at the end of facility training period. These results suggest that accommodative facility training is an efficient method built on loss of symptoms among children with accommodative infacility.

Streff JW, Poynter HL, Jinks B, Wolff B. Changes in achievement scores as a result of a joint optometry and education intervention program. Journal of the American Optometric Association 1990;61:475-81.

This study tested the effect of a visually directed intervention program on changes in standardized test results of intelligence quotient and achievement during kindergarten. Two groups of 19 kindergarten children from equivalent schools were matched for intelligence quotient, age, and sex. Fall and Spring measurements were made in the following areas: intelligence quotient, academic achievement tests, and paper and pencil perceptual tests. A visually based intervention program involving both optometry and education was provided for the experimental group. Kindergarten children in the experimental group who received the visually directed optometry and education intervention program showed significant differences in the rate of change in four of the eight tested areas when matched to the control group.

This "Summary of Research and Clinical Studies" is published with permission from the College of Optometrists in Vision Development. OEP is grateful for the opportunity to include it in this book.

INDEX

BY JANE PAULA PLASS, OD

sports vision, 11, 125–40, 147

squint. *See* strabismus

Stark, Lawrence, 98

"Stereo Sue," vii, 17

strabismus, 20, 24, 37, 95. *See also* esotropia; exotropia; hypertropia

surgery for, 20, 38, 96–97, 111, 159

therapy for, 20, 37–38, 159–60

substance abuse, 77–79. *See also* addiction; drug abuse

suppression, 30–31

T

tachistoscope, 135

telescopic lenses, 122

television, 42–43

Temple Grandin (film), 84

tennis, 127–30, 133, 135–39

Thiagarajan, P., 156

Thinking in Pictures (Grandin), 85–86, 156

Tomlinson, LaDainian, 136

Total Vision (Kavner), vi

TV, 42–43

20/20 is Not Enough, 1st ed. (Seiderman, Marcus, and Hapgood), vi–vii

U

The Ultimate Athlete (Leonard), 133

umpires, 11

The Umpire Strikes Back (Luciano), 125

V

VDT. *See* video display terminals

vergence, 156, 158. *See also* convergence

vertical imbalance, 94, 96–97, 114–15

video display terminals, 42, 98–101, 103. *See also* computer vision syndrome

vision, v–vi, 2–3, 8. *See also* binocular vision

vision and aging, 116–20

Vision and Highway Safety (Allen), 109, 111

vision and learning, 46–48, 51, 57, 69, 72–74, 87, 145–46, 151–52, 154, 158–59, 162– 175. *See also* reading; school—readiness for

vision and personality, 141–44

vision disorders, 2, 10, 19. *See also* binocular vision disorders; refractive errors; specific disorders

age-related, 116–18, 120

case studies, 11–12

diagnosis of, 67–69 (*See also* vision examination)

incidence of, 73

learning disabilities and, 48–49, 73, 84, 146, 150–52

psychological aspects, 80–81

signs and symptoms, 12–14, 55–57, 138–39

types of, 49–51

vision examination, 5–6, 19, 31, 66–67, 74

law and legislation, 92

preschool children and, 34–35

vision screening, 145–46, 165

vision therapy, vii–viii, 3–4, 16–18, 21–25, 48, 96, 105, 151, 155–56, 162, 173

autistic spectrum disorders, 89–90, 156–57

convergence insufficiency, 119, 149–50, 156, 160–61

finding a clinician, 17–18, 23

juvenile delinquents and, 161

low vision and, 123

office-based, 149, 156

older adults and, 116–18, 120

reading and, 63–64, 71, 158–59, 169–74

research, 149–61

sports and, 126–28

strabismus, 38, 159–60

visual acuity, 40, 109, 121, 127

visual attention, 173–74

visual concentration, 137–38

visual demands, 9, 60, 98–99, 103

visual development, 26–29, 31–33, 40–43, 50. *See also* child development

visual field, 109–10, 121

visual imagery, 50

visualization, 135–37

visually aware society, 145–48

visual memory, 167

visual motor integration, 50, 168. *See also* perceptual motor disorders

visual perception, v, 1–2, 7–8, 26–27, 50, 80, 120

visual perception disorders, 51–55, 57, 73

visual reaction time, 112, 118, 134–35

visual skills, 41, 58, 60

visual tracking, 41, 49, 127–28

visual verbal match, 50

vitamins, 34

vocational guidance, 146–47

volleyball, 139

VT. *See* vision therapy